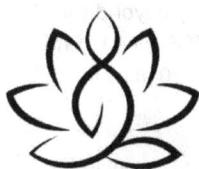

Make Healthy Fit™

Journey Beyond the Plate

7 CLEAR LIFESTYLE PRACTICES™ TO SUSTAINED WEIGHT LOSS

Includes holistic techniques that will *re-awaken* your *spirit* and *nourish* your mind & body

MICHELE JAZZALYN ROSSI

Journey Beyond the Plate
7 Clear Lifestyle Practices™ Proven to End Your Battle with Weight
Copyright © 2018 by Michele J. Rossi

The content of this book is for general informational purposes only. It is not meant to be used, nor should it be used, to diagnose or treat any medical condition or to replace the services of your physician or other healthcare provider. The advice and strategies contained in the book may not be suitable for all readers. Please consult your healthcare provider for any questions that you may have about your own medical situation. Neither the author, publisher, IIN nor any of their employees or representatives guarantees the accuracy of information in this book or its usefulness to a particular reader, nor are they responsible for any damage or negative consequence that may result from any treatment, action taken, or inaction by any person reading or following the information in this book.

Published by Make Healthy Fit, Inc.

ISBN-13: 978-0692125571
ISBN-10: 0692125574

Printed in the United States of America

Cover Design:
Amie Olson, http://promotingnaturalhealth.com

Photography:
Stephanie Bender, https://www.facebook.com/stephanieleaphotography/

Eric Stricko, www.CeresPhotoArt.com

Endorsement

Journey Beyond the Plate is written by Michele J. Rossi, a graduate of the Institute for Integrative Nutrition, where they completed a cutting edge curriculum in nutrition and health coaching taught by the world's leading experts in health and wellness. I recommend you read this book and be in touch with Michele to see how she can help you successfully achieve your goals.

- Joshua Rosenthal, MScEd, Founder/Director, Institute for Integrative Nutrition

Dedication

I dedicate this book to
Ray Szymborski and **Yvonne Szymborski**

Thank you for role-modeling compassion,
a strong work ethic, and responsibility.
Because you encouraged and expected me
to be independent, I learned to climb mountains
and dance in the rain.

The most significant gift in my life
was an extraordinary childhood.

You made our home a happy gathering place
where neighbors, friends, and family were nourished
with exceptional home cooking, unconditional love,
and laughter.

This book is dedicated to you.

I am grateful for the wings you bestowed so that I can fly.

I love you.

Table of Contents

SECTION 1: Introduction   9

Beyond the Plate: 13
The Missing Ingredients to Sustained Weight Loss

Doctor's Ultimatum: 19
Words that Triggered My Transformation

Personal Journey: 25
Heavy and Tired to Awakened and Inspired

SECTION 2: Clear Lifestyle Practices™ to   31
Sustained Weight Loss

Practice #1: CLEAR WHY - Trigger Motivation   35

Practice #2: CLEAR GOALS - Align Compass   45

Practice #3: CLEAR SUPPORT - Nourish Spirit   53

Practice #4: CLEAR PATH - Remove Obstacles   61

Practice #5: CLEAR VISION - Manifest Future   71

Practice #6: CLEAR MIND - Shape Attitude   79

Practice #7: CLEAR CHOICES - Nourish to Flourish   89

Reflection for the Journey Ahead   127

Destined to be Healthy   133

About the Author   135

References   137

Resources   141

Acknowledgments   143

Section 1
Introduction

*"Don't look down at an overweight woman;
instead look up; then ask about her circumstances.
The root cause of poor eating habits is rarely solved
with physical activity and nutrition advice alone."*

- M.J. Rossi

The Missing Ingredients to Sustained Weight Loss

Mary gazed into my eyes, sighed, and said, I've gained back 40 pounds, I'm tired, always hungry, and frustrated with myself. I need help. Can you give me a meal plan? Immediately, I recalled my battle with weight loss. Like Mary, I spent years searching for the elusive, magic diet. Eventually, I discovered the truth about weight management. For this reason, I knew that Mary needed more than food recommendations.

Over the prior ten months, Mary's parents got divorced, her disabled mother moved in, and she became burnt out from a high-pressure job and trying to keep the house in order. Mary was sad, exhausted, and stressed. In the evenings, she turned to comfort food and the couch.

Mary lacked essential foods in life, those that nourish our mind, body, and spirit. She needed to address issues with relationships, career, exercise, and her spiritual outlook. Notably, the circumstances in Mary's life contributed to her poor eating habits. For instance, her stress triggered the production of cortisol, a hormone that put her body into a fight and flight response, aka survival mode. When this occurred, Mary fed her body what she believed it needed to feel better. Because sweet foods trigger the release of dopamine in the brain, a chemical induced feeling of reward, Mary opted for cookies, donuts, and candy. Unfortunately, her temporary sugar high resulted in guilt, fatigue, and more stress. Additionally, she became trapped in a vicious cycle because excess sugar affects her blood sugar level. Consequently, her body produces high levels of insulin which cause fat storage. Then, the body craves another sugar high when blood sugar levels drop. Fact is that sugar is addictive. Mary needed a weight loss recipe that included more ingredients than healthier food and exercise. She needed practices to combat the bodily processes that affected her choices.

The World Health Organization defines health as "a state of complete physical, mental and social well-being and not merely the absence of disease or infirmity."

Unfortunately, the standard advice for shedding pounds is limited to diet and physical activity. Rarely do medical professionals seek to learn the root cause of a patient's weight gain. So, the factors that trigger poor lifestyle habits, such as emotional eating and cravings, are overlooked.

Furthermore, most women deal with stress on a daily basis but are unfamiliar with practices that help to maintain healthy habits while riding life's emotional roller coaster of ups and downs.

Therefore, well-intentioned ladies repeat the same pattern of dieting, weight loss, and weight gain. This recipe persists because of misguided cultural conformity. To put it in another way, a person would never bake the same flavorless cake, each year, and expect it to taste better. That is because baking with known faulty ingredients is not an accepted societal norm. So, it is important to realize that, in general, society continues to reinforce an unsuccessful weight loss recipe.

So, if you have lost and gained weight back, don't feel bad. We live in a fast-paced, over-scheduled, and stressed out culture that is abundant with contradictory information about what foods are good and bad for you.

According to Alexandra Sifferlin, Staff Writer at Time Magazine, the weight loss industry valued at $66.3 billion in 2017; which represents the magnitude of the obesity crisis. To reverse this epidemic, women need to become empowered with knowledge and self-love. In like manner, I redirected my approach to weight loss after a life-threatening condition made me wake-up and realize that dieting was not the answer.

Two years later, I had shed, 115 pounds, and, to-date, have maintained a healthy weight for more than five years. Also, I reversed my insulin resistance, ditched medications for diabetes, blood pressure, and cholesterol, and underwent excess skin removal surgery. Equally important, I reawakened my youthful, vibrant spirit. Then, I returned to school to change careers and become an Integrative Nutrition Health Coach.

I hope to inspire, empower, and guide women to achieve goals that sometimes seem impossible. For this reason, I wrote this book to reveal the missing ingredients needed to Make Healthy Fit and win the battle with weight loss. The journey will empower you with information, choices, flexibility, and permission to stop dieting and celebrate food.

Seven "Clear Lifestyle Practices"™ will guide you on a stimulating journey to self-discovery, a sustainable healthy weight, and happier life. In the first two chapters, you will get a glimpse into my transformational journey. For each of the seven clear lifestyle practices, a worksheet is provided to personalize your plan and shape your unique healthier lifestyle.

*"There are moments that mark your life,
moments when you realize nothing will ever be the same.
And, time is divided into two parts,
before this and after this. "*

- John Hobbes

The Doctor's Ultimatum: Words that Triggered My Transformation

I recall sitting anxiously in a cold examination room when the doctor informed me of the bad news. My blood sugar levels had spiked high above the normal range. Sugar was building up in my blood; therefore, injuring my kidneys and increasing my risk of a heart attack and stroke. Next, the doctor warned me to change my lifestyle, or he would prescribe insulin to control my blood sugar level. Then, I visualized tears rolling down my daughter's cheeks as she worried about losing her single mother. Now, I was frightened and wanted to save my life.

At 50 years-old, I weighed 242 pounds and relied on medications to control high blood sugar, blood pressure, and cholesterol levels. The cluster of these conditions, called Metabolic Syndrome, placed me at high risk for heart attack and stroke.

According to the Center for Disease Control and Prevention, more than one-third of United States adults are obese. And, obesity-related conditions, such as heart disease, diabetes, cancer, and breathing problems, are among the leading causes of premature death. Thus, I had a good reason to fear for my life. However, I did not have suitable food and lifestyle guidance.

My doctor instructed me to avoid white foods, like bagels, potatoes, and bread. However, I did not receive any education about what foods that I should eat. At that time, I did not know that physicians lacked expertise in nutrition. In other words, they do not understand how foods affect your body either positively or negatively. According to David Eisenberg, adjunct associate professor of nutrition at Harvard T.H., "Despite the connection between poor diet and many preventable diseases, only about one-fifth of American medical schools require students to take a nutrition course." Hence, unless a doctor has furthered his or her education in nutrition, the chances are that he or she does not have enough training to provide adequate advice for weight loss. As soon as I learned this fact, I understood why I struggled with obesity and blood sugar control.

For decades, I latched onto the next fad diet because I was confused about what to eat. My food experiments included the Atkins diet, a liquid protein diet, a doctor prescribed meal plan with pills, and a program with hypnosis and a cabinet full of supplements. My success with all these diets was temporary. In fact, most crash diets are less than delicious, eliminate certain foods, and they rarely satisfy hunger. Thus, women often fail to maintain these rigid plans.

I'm not criticizing the Atkins, Jenny Craig, Nutrisystem, or similar diets because some people have success. However, sticking to these plans for a lifetime is challenging. Additionally, people who have relied on these types of prepared foods and supplements may struggle to maintain a healthy weight when they quit the plan. My personal experience down this path led me to choose a different direction.

*"It is in your moments of decision
that your destiny is shaped."*

- Tony Robbins

Initially, I explored healthy lifestyle choices by reading books and scanning credible literature. Unfortunately, I could not lower my blood sugar levels with anything I tried; so, I let go of my ego and engaged a health coach. I did not know it then, but I had taken the first step onto a path that led to an incredible transformation beyond shedding pounds. I was fortunate to have a health coach that role modeled compassion as she challenged a busy, tired, and sick woman to change her lifestyle. Therefore, I am sharing a glimpse into my journey so that you can grasp what you gain when you step onto the path to losing.

"The only journey is the one within."

- Rainer Maria Rilke

My Journey - Heavy and Tired to Awakened and Inspired

"I'm heating up spaghetti, do you want any?" "Yes, Mom," I responded with an amused teenage smile. Once again, she had offered me pasta for an evening snack. At that age, I had no intention of refusing. Healthy was not a word in my vocabulary, and my mother's cooking is exceptional. In fact, my big Italian family has an abundance of cooking talent.

In the 1940s, my great-grandfather, an immigrant from Italy, owned a tap room in Vineland, NJ. People traveled from Philadelphia, PA to eat his cuisine. By the time I was 13 years-old, I could prepare homemade ravioli. At the age of 16, I began working at Zucca's Bakery; where my grandfather baked hundreds of loaves of bread a day.

My grandfather's dad died young; so his mother struggled to feed her eight children. For this reason, he stockpiled food on shelves that spanned the length of his basement; from floor to ceiling. Each time I visited my grandparents, they instructed me to pick out items to take home. I felt blessed to have generous relatives; especially my mom's sister, Dolores.

Every summer, I visited My Aunt and three cousins in Long Island, NY. My week-long stay turned into a non-stop, neighborhood party overflowing with favorite homemade foods. Likewise, I enjoyed food extravaganzas with relatives at the Jersey Shore. Several of my relatives owned beach "shacks" and moved to the Wildwoods for the summer. Multiple families gathered to feast on freshly caught fish, a side of spaghetti, and fresh Italian bread.

In essence, every event in my life revolved around family and food. For two decades, I ate oversized portions; without gaining weight. My ability to stay thin was partly because I ate real meals made with fresh, wholesome ingredients that my body used for energy. I rarely ate boxed foods loaded with sugar, salt, or unrecognizable ingredients and preservatives. Also, I kept fit because of my high activity level.

I played baseball with my brother's friends, jumped rope, rode my bicycle for miles, played recreational volleyball, and twirled a flag in my high school's marching band. My energetic spirit carried over into the arts. Although my hobbies had nothing to do with my weight, I discovered, later, how important they were to my overall well-being.

Mainly, I inherited my father's passion for music and spent hours in my room listening to favorite records. I danced in the basement and enjoyed the occasional concert. My poems filled about one-third of my high school's annual publication, "The Quill." Also, I fell in love with photography during high-school print shop and began developing pictures. Then, I graduated from school, and my lifestyle and health changed dramatically.

I landed a full-time job at a local hospital. In the evenings, I worked a side-hustle as a trained Independent Beauty Consultant; giving women makeovers. Also, I became a DJ playing for a few anniversary parties and weddings. During this time, I remained active by dancing at local clubs every weekend. However, I was so busy that I developed poor eating habits. I lived on popcorn, pizza, ice-cream, and Howard Johnson grand-slam breakfasts. Both, my body and my responsibilities began to grow.

I bought a home at the age of 23, promoted to a Hospital Quality Manager by 28, and one year later became a single mom to a beautiful baby girl. I rarely exercised and struggled to lose my post-pregnancy weight. I spent workdays sitting at a desk; then, driving my daughter to dance class several times a week. This routine spanned from the time my daughter was three-years-old until she could drive herself to dance lessons. To avoid being late for her class, I grabbed take-out burgers and fries and ate in the car.

When I turned 36, I was promoted to a Hospital Department Director and began attending to everyone's needs except my own. I rarely said, "No" to a request for assistance from family, friends, or colleagues. I held volunteer leadership positions at my daughter's school and for several professional organizations. I continued to gain weight and was unaware of the toll it was taking on my health.

By 40-years old, I received a diagnosis of high blood pressure, high-cholesterol, and pre-diabetes. This period in my life is when I experimented with fad diets. Eventually, I got heavier, developed full-blown diabetes, and began taking medications for all three conditions.

By the age of 47, I had landed a Corporate Leadership position. Shortly afterward, I accepted responsibility for coordinating care for my sickly grandfather who became nursing home bound. I was always tired, and my clothes had expanded from a size nine to a twenty. Eventually, I started to fall asleep so suddenly that I felt drugged. Upon developing recurring bronchitis, I finally asked my family for help. Then, I visited the doctor, got the bad news about my health, and took control of my destiny.

Over the next two years, I lost an extraordinary amount of weight; however, what I gained was equally important. I had been obese for so long that I had forgotten how my body was supposed to feel. My energy soared, and I was able to walk long distances without becoming short of breath. Additionally, I stopped snoring, popping antacids for heartburn, and my periodic backaches ceased. At the same time, I re-connected with activities I loved.

I took my camera and favorite music along on walks. Music began to lift my mood and quicken my pace. So, when at home, I started pumping up the sound instead of turning on the television. Music motivated me to get up and clean my house. It entertained me while preparing meals. When a song came on with a great beat, I took a break to dance. Next, I began going to concerts again. When I finally looked back at my unhealthy years, I realized that, like many women, I had lost more than my physical health. I had sacrificed pursuing my interests and desires to serve everyone else.

I had been moving through life; letting it lead me to the next stop. I prioritized everybody's needs over my own, including my employer. I failed to make the time to do the things that nourished my soul. In my youth, I was a poet, a dancer, a photographer, a make-up artist, and a DJ. The spirit of that woman had become dormant. When I started attending concerts again, dancing, and taking photos, I leaped from happy to joyful. I had believed that my overweight body was the problem, but, now I know it was my mindset.

"Weight loss can change your whole character. That always amazed me: Shedding pounds does change your personality. It changes your philosophy of life because you recognize that you are capable of using your mind to change your body."

- Jean Nidetch

In 2013, just when I believed that I was self-aware, I had to submit to a battery of self-discovery tests during my first course back in college. The purpose of the testing was to guide students to their best career path. My results indicated that I was artistic, social, and enterprising. My career recommendations were Music Director, Choreographer, Stage Manager, Coach, Teacher, and Religious Worker.

I had no idea when I stepped onto a new path to lose weight and avoid insulin that it would lead me to my destiny, serving others as a health coach. You don't need to know how your journey will end. Just take the first step and never give up.

Now, let us start working on your personalized recipe for sustained weight loss.

Section 2
Clear Lifestyle Practices™
to Sustained Weight Loss

*"People often say that motivation doesn't last.
Well, neither does bathing
- that's why we recommend it daily."*

- Zig Ziglar

Clear Lifestyle Practice #1
Clear Why: Trigger Motivation

Remember Mary, the woman who asked me to give her a meal plan. Mary is a fictitious character; however, she represents numerous women who have talked to me about their desire to lose weight. So, I will call upon Mary to demonstrate significant points, such as your "Clear Why" necessary to trigger self-motivation.

Following my initial interaction with Mary, we formally met, in my office, to discuss her health concerns and goals. Once again, Mary tells me that she is overweight, tired, and frustrated with herself. So, I ask her, "Is losing weight something you think you should do, want to do, or need to do?" Mary immediately responds, "My doctor says my numbers are just fine, and my husband doesn't care how much I weigh. I don't need to lose weight, but I know that I should be healthier. Perhaps, I won't be as tired. Please, just tell me what to eat so I won't have to figure it out on my own."

After speaking with Mary for an hour, she realized that lifestyle changes, beyond food, were necessary to achieve her weight loss goal. Even so, I knew that her motivation level might weaken. Mary did not have the "Clear Why" that is essential to withstand the inevitable obstacles on her path to a 40-pound loss. Specifically, Mary felt like she should get healthy, but she did not feel it was necessary.

According to the world's leading high-performance coach, Brendon Burchard, *"When you have high necessity, you strongly agree with this statement, I feel deep emotional drive and commitment to succeeding, and it consistently forces me to work hard, stay disciplined, and push myself."*

With this in mind, it is essential for a woman to get clear on why losing weight is necessary. Then, she can begin to re-shape her lifestyle. To get clear, a women must dig deep into her soul and be honest about the "real" need for shedding pounds. Notably, physical appearance; not health may be the real catalyst.

When I decided to transform my health, I did not understand the magnitude of this essential lifestyle practice. I progressed toward my goal, but it took an extraordinary encounter with a Rock Star to re-kindle my inner spirit and spark the birth of my "Clear Why." This pivotal interaction altered my thinking and motivation level.

My initial why was huge. I feared depending on insulin, nursing home care, and leaving my young daughter parentless. But, the idea of a significant lifestyle change seemed daunting. After all, how could, I, a busy, sick, corporate healthcare leader find the time to exercise, cook, and learn how to manage my diabetes. And, the thought of giving up pizza made me sad.

Perhaps you can understand my former doubting attitude. Have you ever put off losing weight because you dreaded feeling hungry, going to the gym, or listening to family members complain about junk foods suddenly disappearing from the pantry? If that is so; then you are not alone.

Women tend to delay prioritizing their health because they perceive that the path ahead will be difficult and unpleasant. In reality, being overweight is uncomfortable and challenging. Most women who carry excess weight tend to experience one or more of the following issues:

- Lack of energy or fatigue
- Difficulty breathing when walking
- Indigestion or heartburn
- Pain from joint stress or inflammation
- Feeling uncomfortable with body image
- Snoring
- Inadequate or poor sleep
- Struggling to fit into attractive looking clothes

The list above contains excellent reasons to want to lose weight; however, these weight loss "whys" rarely lead to sustained motivation. A "Clear Why" must be robust enough that failing is not an option. For example, most women get a job to pay for living expenses. Even if their work environment is unpleasant, they faithfully show up because money is necessary to cover bills.

Similarly, a weight loss motivator is one that drives you to show up and succeed; even on unpleasant days. For that reason, I have included a worksheet to guide you to discover your "Clear Why." But before you move forward, I am sharing the experience that changed my attitude from doubtful to determined. I hope that by revealing my story, you will better understand the importance of your own why.

The moment started with these words: "You! You! You are Miss America!"

My heart was pounding, and I was catching my breath after getting lost in dance to the pounding rhythm of Styx's famous song, Miss America. I heard a man screaming. I looked up and realized it was Styx's front man, Tommy Shaw. He was kneeling on the edge of an outdoor stage; his arm extended, finger pointed at me, and shouting You! You! You are Miss America! I stood, in the first row directly under Tommy Shaw's microphone, in a daze.

When my brain fog lifted, I realized what had transpired and flashed a childish smile at Tommy. I did not know it immediately, but he had given me a gift, my life-changing "Clear Why."

Earlier that day, on my 51st birthday, I boarded a train to experience the Taste of DC and to celebrate my weight loss progress. I still had 60 pounds to lose and struggled with self-doubt, plateaus, and the reality of sagging excess skin.

After I arrived home, something magical happened. I discovered a compelling and positive reason for achieving my goals. Instead of focusing on weight loss to avoid insulin and prevent further illness, I focused on everything I would gain. To put it differently, I stopped focusing on the negative reasons for improving my health. Consequently, my motivation and determination became unstoppable. Heck, I was Miss America.

I had lost 55 pounds in one year; my blood sugars were stable, and, I rocked my body so hard that I caught the attention of a Rock Star. Suddenly, I remembered the healthier version of me, the energetic dancer with an hour-glass shape who looked and felt sexy. Tommy Shaw did not spot an obese woman in the crowd; instead, he witnessed the inner spirit of a woman whose hips, feet, and arms shifted rapidly in sync with the rhythm of the band's music.

Later, I discovered that Tommy Shaw had conquered addictions with drugs and alcohol. If the man who told me that I was Miss America was Mr. America himself, then I planned to be a role model for others too. I needed to melt the remaining layers of fat off my body and show up at the next concert looking like Miss America. Like Justin Timberlake, I planned to bring sexy back!

From that point forward, whenever, I felt too tired to exercise or became tempted to grab junk food, I grasped my "Clear Why" and kicked my tired butt off the couch.

"In everyone's life, at some time, our inner fire goes out. It is then burst into flame by an encounter with another human being. We should all be thankful for those people who rekindle the inner spirit."

- Albert Schweitzer

A "Clear Why" becomes a woman's solid arrow aimed at her health goals. It is her unique weapon that continually helps defend against self-doubt, fatigue, temptation, poor attitude, lack of motivation, and setbacks.

Three important points:

1. A woman does not need a rock star, a lover, a friend, or anyone else to recognize the vibrant spirit within her. She can re-kindle her spirit by deciding who she wants to be; then believing in herself

2. An overweight woman may be loved and desired by her partner, but it is important that she feels healthy, comfortable, and desirable

3. As a woman ages, she may change her weight loss goal; however, she will always need a "Clear Why" to hit the new bullseye

A "Clear Why" also serves as a cheerleader throughout a woman's transformational journey. For this reason, I asked my client, Mary, to re-think her why until she knew why losing weight was necessary for her well-being.

Then, I had Mary create a mental image of herself standing confidently at the entrance of a pathway that led to a lighter and healthier body.

Now, picture yourself on a new path; ready to embark on your weight loss journey. You are equipped with your Clear Why to remind you why you started.

CLEAR WHY WORKSHEET

Is losing weight something you need or something that you think you should do? If you don't believe weight loss is necessary; then why is it a goal? _____

_____

_____

_____

If you need to lose weight, why? I need to achieve my goal because _____

_____

_____

_____

How will you benefit? I will (feel / look / act / be able to) _____

_____

_____

_____

What is your current motivation level? On a scale of 1-5, with one being low and five being high, my motivation level is: _____

Reaching your goal(s) should be a positive journey, but the road may be long and bumpy. Recalling your "Clear Why" helps to sustain motivation. If your motivation level scored 3 or lower; then ask yourself, if I don't do this now, will I regret it forever?

If so, why_____

_____

_____

_____

My CLEAR WHY is:

_____

_____

_____

_____

_____

_____

*"All successful people have a goal.
No one can get anywhere unless he knows
where he wants to go and what he wants to do."*

- Norman Vincent Peale

Clear Lifestyle Practice #2
Clear Goals: Align Compass

Mary dug deep into her emotions to determine why she needed to lose weight. As a result, she decided to take more responsibility for her health. Now, she was eager to learn how to achieve success instead of waiting for a list of acceptable meals. Accordingly, I asked Mary what path she intended to take to her desired weight.

Like a GPS that directs our travel, Mary needed "Clear Goals" to guide her journey to weight loss. I encouraged her to write down the number of pounds she wanted to lose; then, forget about her body size. Instead, I encouraged Mary to establish primary goals that would make weight loss happen, such as adding in fruits and vegetables, eating smaller portions of sweets, and increasing physical activity. To emphasize, the number of pounds she needed to lose became a mere data point to assess progress towards improving health.

In general, people are told to diet when health issues surface. Unfortunately, we are conditioned to believe that by losing weight we get healthy. Fact is, we shed fat and keep it off as an outcome of improved health. Additionally, body size is not an indication of health. For example, a woman can be skinny and malnourished because of an eating disorder. Furthermore, women tend to feel disappointed when weight loss is slow. First thing to remember, every step forward moves you closer to your goal.

Another misconception about setting goals is that you stop when you achieve them. Just like a game of archery, you would not stop playing the game once you hit the bullseye. Nor would someone stop vacationing at the beach because they've traveled there in the past. A goal is something that you aim to achieve and maintain. You continue to practice and play. Eventually, you miss less because the game becomes easier. That is to say, you cannot sustain weight loss if you stop playing once you lose. With this in mind, the 7 Clear Lifestyle Practices revealed in this book are intended for you to apply as often as needed.

Now, for a moment, picture Mary who is still standing at the entrance of her pathway and feeling empowered. She gazes straight ahead and visualizes a large, bright archery target. Her goals are clearly displayed. She recalls her Clear Why; then, points her mind's arrow directly at her "Clear Goals." She accepts that her thoughts will occasionally point in the wrong direction; away from the target. In fact, that is how the game of healthy lifestyle is played. You give yourself permission to enjoy food and life. Some days you eat salad and some days you eat a cupcake. But, you keep aiming for the bullseye because failure is not an option.

Comparatively, the only time I thought about my weight was during my monthly accountability check-in with my health coach. Instead, I committed to the goals that made weight loss happen. For example, I skipped the bread at parties so that I could have a piece of cake. If I became hungry near dinner time, I ate an apple to keep me full so that I had time to cook. Thus, instead of satisfying my ravenous appetite with take out junk food, I enjoyed a delicious healthy meal.

Given these points, do not be afraid to set challenging goals. A close friend advised me to lower my expectations because my weight loss goal was too aggressive for my age. Proudly, I blew past my goal by six pounds. In like manner, be careful not to let anyone's opinion limit your own beliefs.

"All who have accomplished great things have had a great aim, have fixed their gaze on a goal which was high, one which sometimes seemed impossible."

- Orison Swett Marden

Fortunately, my health coach prompted me to write down goals; otherwise, I would have had vague dreams circling around in my head. My initial goal was to lower my blood sugar level. By achieving this target, I dropped a couple of dress sizes. In six months, I had lost 20 pounds and without increasing my physical activity level. Notably, small steps turn into big ones. It is important to realize that you do not have to start every goal at once. My two year journey, to drop 115 pounds, felt like forever. Now, looking back, it seems more like a second in my life. Slow and steady changes aid in forming long-term, sustainable habits.

Equally important, goals need to be specific, measurable, attainable, realistic, and time-based. A healthy weight loss goal is one to two pounds per week; depending on a woman's starting body size. With this in mind, Mary established short and long-term goals that met this criteria. She wrote down, I will lose four pounds per month; achieving a 40 pound weight loss over ten months. "Clear Goals" must be simple to understand. One way to make them clear is to use the widely accepted SMART acronym. Below are examples of how to apply the SMART acronym to define short and long-term goals.

SMART GOAL EXAMPLES

SPECIFIC: *Not too general*

BAD EXAMPLE:	Get in Shape
GOOD EXAMPLE:	Lose 40 pounds

MEASURABLE: *Something you can track*

BAD EXAMPLE:	Increase Physical Activity
GOOD EXAMPLE:	Walk 30 minutes a day

ATTAINABLE: *Something that is doable, but not to easy*

BAD EXAMPLE:	Quit all sugar
GOOD EXAMPLE:	Eliminate soda and reduce sugar in my coffee to 1 tsp.

REALISTIC: *Something that is real rather than ideal*

BAD EXAMPLE:	Hire a personal chef to make my meals
GOOD EXAMPLE:	Eat a side-salad with dinner 4 nights a week

TIME-BASED: *A date for long-term goal or time increments for short-term goals*

    BAD EXAMPLE: Go to bed earlier

    GOOD EXAMPLE: Go to bed and get up 1 hour earlier every day

Although Mary preferred to arrive at her destination quickly, she chose a steady stroll. She knew that small steps would be enjoyable and sustainable; unlike a challenging high-speed run.

CLEAR GOALS WORKSHEET

PRIMARY (Long & short-term goals that make weight loss happen)

1. _____

_____

_____

This goal is: *Specific, Measurable, Attainable, Realistic, and Time-based*

2. _____

_____

_____

This goal is: *Specific, Measurable, Attainable, Realistic, and Time-based*

3. _____

_____

_____

This goal is: *Specific, Measurable, Attainable, Realistic, and Time-based*

SECONDARY (Weight loss goal)

1. _____

_____

_____

*"Surround yourself with good people
who encourage and love you.
There are always ups and downs,
no matter how successful you are."*

- Liana Liberato

Clear Lifestyle Practice #3
Clear Support: Nourish Spirit

Once Mary and I finalized her remaining goals, I asked if her friends and family would be supportive of her lifestyle changes. She shrugged her shoulders and sighed. Mary's husband, Pete, encouraged her to do what she wanted, but said that he loved her as is. Regrettably, Mary anticipated complaints from Pete. He had become accustomed to take out burgers, cheesesteaks, and pizza. Although Pete was overweight, he was not ready to make a personal change. Also, Mary anticipated ridicule from her co-workers who indulged in donuts, cookies, and candy on a daily basis. Lastly, Mary had disconnected from friends after she started caring for her mother. Considering those circumstances, I asked Mary who she knew that enjoyed a healthy lifestyle. I suggested that she reconnect with them.

Fact is, not all family members and friends will be able to support you in the way that you need. Unfortunately, their good intentions may become overshadowed by unintentional, disrespectful behaviors. For example, your partner may bring home a box of donuts and continue to offer them to you; even after you've declined. Or, a friend will abruptly change the conversation when you mention a new healthy recipe. Also, children may complain when an abundance of cookies, candy, and chips disappear from the pantry. Furthermore, as other female friends and family members notice your new thinner body, they might become jealous of your success. You become a reminder of their personal battle with weight.

If you let it, these type of sarcastic comments and unsupportive behaviors can be emotionally wounding. In addition, it may weaken your commitment to avoid the unpleasant feedback. It is important to realize that when you change your lifestyle, you are affecting the people around you; especially those who live with you. To gain "Clear Support" it is necessary to establish clear communication with your partner and other significant people in your life.

One way to relay your needs without putting someone on the defense is to speak with "I" statements instead of "You" statements. An "I" statement allows you to express your feelings respectfully. For instance, "I feel like I'm not able to fit in time for my workout and it's making me upset. Can we talk about how to work this out?" A "You" statement often sounds blameful and disrespectful. For example, "You are not supporting me or doing anything around the house that you promised. So, I missed my workout, again."

As women, we tend to put ourselves last. We are caregivers who need to learn to say, "No," ask for help, and put ourselves first. Even on airplanes, the attendants instruct parents to put on their oxygen mask first. We cannot be our best for others if we don't care for ourselves.

*"I define connection as the energy that exists between people
when they feel seen, heard, and valued;
when they can give and receive without judgment;
and when they derive sustenance and strength
from the relationship."*

- Brené Brown

Additionally, communicating your intentions to the people in your circle helps to keep you accountable to your goals. The bottom line is that you cannot blame others for your choices. Frankly, you are devaluing yourself and sending a clear message to them that you are not committed. When people realize that you are serious, they may become more supportive and respectful of your needs.

To clarify, lack of support and hurtful behaviors can become obstacles on the path to your goals. Do not underestimate the need for support to maintain a positive mindset. According to the American Psychological Association, "Lifestyle Changes are a Process. Accepting help from those who care about you and will listen strengthens your resilience and commitment."

Like Mary, I chose a health coach, Shannon, to be one of my key supports. Shannon did not judge my path, ridicule my choices, or attempt to hinder my progress. Instead, she lifted me, challenged me, and enlightened me with knowledge and guidance. I did not anticipate the rude communications from my friends. By focusing on myself, I had less time to spend with other people. Once, I was asked, "Are you getting too pretty for us now?" I ignored the question. Hence, I offered this advice to Mary, "Be kind to unkind people because they need it the most."

I recommended that Mary complete the Clear Support Worksheet. A week later, she sent me a text decorated with multiple smile emojis. The friends that she had contacted were happy that she reached out to them and felt honored to help her.

"My path gets more beautiful when you walk it with me."

- Toni Sorenson

CLEAR SUPPORT WORKSHEET

The "Clear Support" Worksheet is intended to help you select the person or persons who will cheer you on, celebrate successes, and hold you accountable when you are hurdling plateaus, relationship changes, and other obstacles on your path.

When selecting a support person or persons, consider what you already know about the personalities of your family, friends, and co-workers. Then, get clear about who will live up to the roles below: One person may serve in all these roles.

1. **The person or persons who will attentively listen and look forward to hearing about my progress, obstacles, and success:**

    _____

2. **The person or persons who might lend a hand so that I can prioritize my health:**

    _____

3. **The person or persons who is like-minded and will enjoy talking about health foods, recipes, etc.**

    _____

4. **If I begin to feel overwhelmed or unable to achieve my goals, I will seek support to ensure my success. The best option for me and my lifestyle is:**

    _____

If you answered no to question #4, then re-think you "Clear Why."

"The mark of a great man is one who knows when to set aside the important thing in order to accomplish the vital ones."

- Brandon Sanderson

Clear Lifestyle Practice #4
Clear Path: Remove Obstacles

Mary felt ready to implement her goals and experience a lighter, healthier, and energetic body. However, she did not realize that the path ahead was cluttered. For one thing, Mary still faced the issues that hindered her success in the past. She worked long hours and took sole responsibility for the care of her disabled mother.

I predicted that Mary would take a few steps forward and either stumble, get stuck, or quit the journey. Failure to achieve goals is common because women neglect to prioritize their needs. Instead, they continue to concentrate on the needs and wants of other people. Far to often, women fail to set boundaries because they feel obligated, helpless, or guilty saying, "No."

It is important to realize that communicating your needs is not the same as making time to address those needs. For example, one of Mary's goals was to cook at home more often. In the past, she relied on the convenience of fast food for dinner because of her late work schedule. Thus, I asked Mary how she planned to address these barriers.

A "Clear Path," requires eliminating or fixing the situations placed ahead of your own goals. To achieve a healthy weight and body, you need to schedule the time to develop new eating habits, a fitness program, and other self-care practices.

Thus, actions are necessary to remove the obstacles that will interfere with your progress. Think about a time when you planned a vacation. What arrangements did you make for the trip to be a success? Perhaps, you requested time off from work, made reservations, secured a pet sitter, or serviced your vehicle. Similar to a vacation, you must plan for the journey. Before my doctor warned me that I might need Insulin, I believed that eating less food and eliminating sweets was sufficient to transform my health.

Fortunately, I became wise enough to realize that I needed to prioritize me. So, my efforts went beyond the plate to achieve success. For instance, I had been visiting my grandfather in a nursing home five times a week and staying there for three hours.

Instead, I limited my future visits to one hour. Furthermore, I stopped spending dozens of weekends babysitting or assisting family and friends with resumes and other paperwork.

That being said, I failed to address all the obstacles on my path, including my excuses for not exercising. In fact, it took my health coach, Shannon, to challenge me. "NO, I'm too busy, I exclaimed! My drive to work takes more than an hour, my job is demanding, I eat lunch at my desk, and spend two hours driving home in bumper-to-bumper traffic. And, I'm cooking more often." Ugh, I thought. Doesn't Shannon understand how busy I am? Seriously, how much more can I handle? I'm exhausted after dinner. All I want to do is plop my overweight and tired butt on the recliner to relax and watch TV. But, Shannon strongly recommended that I make the time to walk for 10 minutes during my lunch break. After I hung up the phone, I came to grips with the fact that my boss never told me to skip my legally required breaks. I had chosen to prioritize my workload over my health. Conversely, if my employer expected me to forego lunch, I would have reached out to human resources for support. Subsequently, I set boundaries between my professional and home life. Over time, I increased the length of my walks.

Six months after that awkward conversation with my health coach, I became addicted to walking because it developed into pleasurable "me time." I continue to enjoy four-mile walks; several times a week. Walking in nature clears my mind, and, sometimes, I dream while walking through the serene neighborhood park. Also, I reap energy through the beat of my favorite music when tackling inclines on the gym's treadmill.

I discovered that physical activity aided in weight loss; especially when shedding those last few challenging pounds. Equally exciting, I observed my legs became thin and firm. If I had kept making excuses, my important goals would have remained a dream.

*"When I complain about how busy I am, it is as if someone
put all these things on my plate without my approval.
When in fact, I make my life the way it is.
I chose to be in school. I chose to work three jobs.
I chose to pack my weeks with plans and travel whenever
possible. The question is: Is it all worth it?
If it is, be grateful and proud of everything you do.
If it's not, make a change."*

- Megan Wycklendt

Another critical point is that no amount of motivation and good intentions will prevent your failure. Lifestyle change requires empowered choices that can be difficult and emotional to implement. A "Clear Path" necessitates that you promote yourself to Boss and begin to lead your life in the direction of your goals and dreams. When you begin to make an excuse, remember that is your job to eliminate the problem or seek help to fix it. Harmony in life is absent when you fail to focus on the goals that you deem necessary.

*"The most important reason for your "no"
is that you need your downtime so you won't behave like a jerk
because you're depleted. And you don't want to battle
an appetite spiked by the stress of over commitment.
But that's your secret; others don't need that information.
So just smile, say no, thank you, and keep moving."*

- Holly Mosier

Once Mary successfully carved out the time to implement her goals, I told her that she still had "mind work" to do before stepping onto her path.

CLEAR PATH WORKSHEET

Complete the worksheet below to identify; then mitigate the obstacles along your path to success. Consider how you can eliminate or fix them.

The template below includes prompts to help you think about areas of your life that you may need to change:

1. **Involvement in volunteer activities or clubs:** What events could you remove from your schedule? How are they serving your life? Are these activities more important than your health goals?

    I plan to:

    _____

    _____

2. **Commitments made to family or friends:** Can these commitments be shared or served by someone else? Can these commitments, such as babysitting, be time-limited?

    I plan to:

    _____

    _____

3. **Work Schedule:** Does your job or other personal schedules routinely prohibit you from eating lunch? Do you regularly work extended hours? How can you take charge of your life to make changes; even minor ones to free up time?

    I plan to:

    _____

    _____

4. **Technology:** Can you limit the time you spend with technology? Consider setting boundaries, such as limiting your time on social media and watching only a few favorite television shows?

   I plan to:

   _____

   _____

5. **Relationships:** Are you spending time with people who drain your energy because of their negativity? Can you reduce the amount of time I spent with them or walk away from toxic relationships gracefully?

   I plan to:

   _____

   _____

6. **Other:** What other activities and commitments have you made that are not necessary? If they bring you joy; then consider keeping them or limiting your time. If they stress you, remove or fix them.

   I plan to:

   _____

   _____

*"If you can't imagine the future,
you can't possibly create it."*

- Wolf Management Consultants

Clear Lifestyle Practice #5
Clear Vision: Manifest Future

By the time of our next appointment, Mary had successfully addressed four Clear Lifestyle Practices to apply throughout her life's journey. She was equipped with her Clear Why to trigger motivation, Clear Goals to serve as a compass, Clear Support to nourish her spirit, and a Clear Path to enable success. Even so, Mary was weighed down by limiting beliefs. Her past failures generated doubt about what is possible. To put it another way, Mary could not to see beyond the reality of her eyes. She kept saying that she would be happy to lose 20 pounds. Although her goal was reasonable, Mary could not imagine her future self 40 pounds lighter. She had to vision a new reality based on what she wished to see; instead of dwelling in her present beliefs.

A Clear-Vision is an image of your desired future. It is a mental picture of your enhanced body and lifestyle. Perhaps, you see a slender woman wrapped in fashionable clothes or a fit lady walking confidently into a party. Often, this mental image connects to your "Clear-Why." For instance, if your Clear Why is re-gaining the ability to participate in a sport that you once loved; then you might vision yourself swimming or riding a bicycle.

Throughout my health and career transformation, I created a Clear Vision for my future. I am sharing those mental pictures with you as examples of how to manifest the life of your dreams.

- While losing weight, I imagined my body with hourglass curves and toned arms and legs. I also pictured myself dancing without losing breathe.

- When I achieved those goals and discovered my life's purpose, I visioned walking away from my corporate career to serve as a full-time health coach. Ironically, the day after I left my job, I observed a social media post that read, she is living the life that she imagined. I held back the happy tears.

- My current vision is a "zen life" with meaningful work. I see myself living in a new home with a dedicated fitness room and a large kitchen. I am blissfully preparing healthy meals while sipping on a small glass of fine wine. I have mastered yoga. I travel to Italy often and have learned to make incredible meals by taking cooking classes with the most excellent chefs.

- Lastly, I imagine that my work as a health coach, author, and advocate has contributed to a reversal of the obesity and diabetes epidemics across the nation by helping women live happy and healthy lives. I picture myself speaking to organizations responsible for making changes in the healthcare system and educating large audiences of women.

Another way to keep your goals and desires top of the mind is to create a vision board. This is a collage of images, notes, or quotes to display for your two eyes to see and implant into your mind. The intent is to select items that will trigger a pleasant feeling and inspire you. Here are some tips for developing the board:

- Select one large framed cork or poster board or multiple small boards.

- Choose multiple images from photographs, magazines, drawings, or cards. Based on your preference, leave space in-between the pictures or overlap them.

- Establish a mood for completing this activity. Decide if you want to work on the board alone or with friends or family. If you work on your board alone, consider listening to music that connects with your emotions. If you do this with a group, serve healthy treats and delight in examining everyone's masterpiece.

- Display the vision board in a room where you spend the most time.

What we pay attention to manifests in our life. For instance, when I decided that my next car would be a Nissan Altima, I began to see an abundance of those vehicles on the road. Two years later, I visited a dealership. The add-ons that I wanted for the car were out of my price range. However, my feelings were so connected to what I had imagined that I bickered with management for six hours. Eventually, I purchased the car of my dreams and within budget. That is to say; I refused to give up because, in my mind, that exact car was already mine.

In summary, mental images can inspire you to do what you need to do to reach your goals instead of doing what you want to do. Specifically, when you routinely see an image of your future self, you are more likely to exercise than watch television.

*"Your vision will become clear only when you look
into your heart. Who looks outside dreams.
Who looks inside, awakens."*

- Anonymous

Thus, I told Mary to think about two things every time she faces a choice in life, such as what to eat or whether to work out. First, she should recall her Clear Why to remember why she started; and, second, her Clear Vision to see what is at stake based on her decision. Moreover, I reminded Mary to call her support person when struggles, such as plateaus, stress, or a tragedy, affect her emotional state.

During difficult times in life, the most determined woman may need external motivation to stay on track or remain positive when she misses the bullseye for an extended period. I reminded Mary that all long journeys consist of rest stops and wrong turns. The important thing is to find your way back to the path that leads to your beautiful destination.

CLEAR VISION WORKSHEET

Complete the worksheet below to identify images that will generate positive emotions and lift your spirit. Then, vision these mental pictures every day; especially when you are not motivated to act on your goals. If desired, create a vision board to display these same images.

1. **Images connected to my "Clear Why" are:**

   _____

   _____

   _____

   _____

2. **Other Images that will trigger pleasant feelings and motivate and inspire me are:**

   _____

   _____

   _____

   _____

   _____

   _____

   _____

   _____

   _____

   _____

"If you are not taking responsibility for your state of consciousness, you are not taking responsibility for life."

- Eckhart Tolle

Clear Lifestyle Practice #6
Clear Mind: Shape Attitude

I welcomed Mary with a hug and a big smile when she entered my office. Finally, I was ready to give her the same gift that an enlightened friend shared with me. This present did not cost me anything, but the value to Mary would be transformative to her success and happiness. Immediately, I told Mary I had a present for her. Then, like a child with a secret, I whispered "It's all in your head."

"Every thought we think is creating our future."

- Louise Hay

A "Clear Mind" requires using your mind as a tool to master your life. Surprisingly, many men and women do not realize how their thoughts influence their feelings, actions, and destiny. For instance, say a woman wants to join a fitness center, but she worries about people staring and judging her body size. As a result, she forgoes the gym and misses an opportunity for free, professional help. In this situation, the woman's thoughts are controlling her actions. Thus, she is paving her destiny by giving up an activity that would expedite weight loss and tone her body.

Additionally, these kind of thoughts are assumptive and make women feel bad about themselves. Yes, someone can exercise at home; however, the point is that negative thoughts prevent you from doing what you need or want to do.

> *"Care about what other people think*
> *and you will always be their prisoner."*
>
> - Lao Tzu

The most compelling evidence that your mind can be a friend or an enemy is my observations during the last five years. As a slim woman, I frequently see overweight females staring at me while I workout. These ladies are unaware that I formerly weighed 242 pounds. For this reason, I typically walk up to a gazer, introduce myself, and tell them my story. I make this effort to inspire hope and create awareness that many people in the fitness center did not arrive there healthy. In reality, gym members who glance at an obese woman are more inclined to silently cheer her on than form an opinion. Thus, become mindful of any negative thoughts that emotionally weigh you down. Then, purposefully shift them to something positive.

To further demonstrate, did you ever feel like walking away from someone who constantly complains or thrives on drama? These are people who turn negative thoughts into words. Subsequently, their character is formed as a person to avoid. Unfortunately, this individual's destiny is likely to be alone, lonely, or surrounded by a tribe of miserable friends.

My explanations resonated with Mary and triggered her

to realize how many complainers occupied her office. Thus, she immediately began to think positively about her work and life situation. She also realized that she may need to find new employment if her manager did not agree to reduce her hours. Mary had gained the gift of mental power to shape her attitude; regardless of her circumstances.

"Whatever we plant in our subconscious mind and nourish with repetition and emotion will one day become a reality."

- Earl Nightingale

The key is to become aware of your feelings. I encouraged Mary to let go of past disappointments and hurts because she could not change the past. I explained that worrying about the future is like wishing for what she does not want to have happen. Explicitly, Mary would have a difficult time acting on her weight loss goals if she maintained a pessimistic attitude and maintained limiting beliefs. Negative thoughts create stress; which can lead to overeating, anxiety, depression, and dysfunction.

To clarify, living positively does not mean that you cannot grieve or feel pain. But, it does mean that you have the power to shift you thoughts, rise from distress, shine your light, and shape your destiny. People who practice controlling their thoughts create happier, healthier, and successful lives because they become resilient. A point often overlooked is that health includes mental, physical, and social well-being. Notably, a journey to sustained weight loss must go beyond the plate to direct your decision making tool, the mind.

"Watch your thoughts, they become words;
watch your words, they become actions;
watch your actions, they become habits;
watch your habits, they become character;
watch your character, for it becomes your destiny."

- Frank Outlaw

Ultimately, Mary felt confident in her ability to lose 40 pounds. She understood the importance of using her mind as a tool to influence her choices. Next, I recommended that Mary develop at least one mindfulness practice using the Clear Mind Worksheet. At the same time, I provided her with handouts for our next discussion on Clear Choices related to food, physical activity, and sleep.

CLEAR MIND WORKSHEET

Reflective and spiritual practices help to quiet and clear the mind. They also aid in concentration, awareness, and focus. This Clear Mind Worksheet includes a brief description of four leading complementary and integrative practices. However, it is not meant to be a comprehensive list of practices, instructions, or benefits. The purpose of this activity is to suggest techniques to enhance the interconnectedness of your mind, body, and spirit.

I encourage you to experiment with one or more of these practices. Give yourself time to realize the benefits before judging the effectiveness. If an approach doesn't work for you, consider selecting an alternative.

MEDITATION

The four common features of meditation include:

1. Selecting a quiet area with little to no distractions

2. Lying or sitting down in a comfortable position

3. Focusing on the pattern of your breath, a word, or phrase

4. Acknowledging distractive thoughts; then letting them go

According to the National Center for Complementary and Integrative Health, "Some research suggests that meditation may physically change the brain and body and could potentially help to improve many health problems and promote healthy behaviors."

YOGA

Approaches to yoga vary; however, the practice is typically experienced through a combination of breathing techniques and body postures.

According to the Yoga Alliance, this practice is used to "help raise their quality of life in such diverse areas as fitness, stress relief, wellness, vitality, mental clarity, healing, peace of mind and spiritual growth."

JOURNALING

Like meditation, this practice helps with focus, awareness, and mental clarity. You can journal in a variety of ways. The list below represents three common techniques:

1. **Food Diary:** A daily log of foods can help identify eating patterns and the emotions connected with your choices. For instance, when you notice that you have consumed junk foods, write down how you felt that day. Once you realize the trigger, you are more likely to make a mindful choice the next time.

2. **Gratitude:** A daily list of things, situations, or people that you are grateful to have in your life. This exercise helps you to focus on the positive; thus shaping your attitude for the day. The notes can be as simple as expressing thanks for the sunshine or a milestone that you reached along your journey to a healthy weight.

3. **Free-flow Writing:** A blank piece of paper filled with words or phrases that capture your daily intentions, goals, thoughts, ideas, or plans, such as self-care, recreation,

hobbies, etc. Write with abandon; without editing.

According to Health Fitness Revolution " All of your thoughts, dreams, and worries swirl around in your head. It's good to sometimes sit still and think things through, but other times you need to focus. Journaling lets you channel the background noise onto paper so that your brain can problem-solve the here and now issues."

PRAYER

Similar to the benefits of expressing gratitude, people who believe in a higher power are more likely to elicit positive emotions. In essence, their faith acknowledges influence over their life; bringing about a sense of comfort and hope.

According to Psychology Today, one of the five scientifically proven benefits of prayer is self-control. "Activities that require self-control are fatiguing, making it more difficult to make good choices the more you have to use your "self-control muscle." Think about it. You are more likely to lose your cool or engage in mindless eating when you are mentally exhausted."

I plan to develop or maintain a mindfulness practice, such as meditation, yoga, journaling, or prayer by:

_____

_____

_____

_____

"Health is a relationship between you and your body"

- Terri Guillemets

Clear Lifestyle Practice #7
Clear Choices: Nourish to Flourish

Ten minutes past Mary's appointment time, I reached for my phone to send her a text. Simultaneously, she burst through my office door and twirled across the room. Then, Mary stood tall, flashed a broad smile and announced, "I've lost three pounds and joined the gym." As we clapped a loud "high-five," I witnessed a beautiful twinkle in her eyes. Eagerly, I asked, "What changes did you make in your lifestyle?" Proudly, Mary said, I did what you recommended. I thought about why I wanted to lose weight and talked myself into cooking dinner at least six nights a week. On Fridays, Pete and I plan to enjoy our favorite pizza.

Intuitively, Mary knew that home cooked meals are healthier than take-out options. Even so, she looked forward to guidance about food options. In light of Mary's decision to join a fitness center, I introduced the remaining Clear Lifestyle Practice that is fundamental to weight loss and overall well-being.

Clear Choices is the most challenging practice because it typically requires lifestyle change in the areas of food, physical activity, and sleep. For this reason, all of the preceding Clear Lifestyle Practices are intended to prepare and strengthen your mind, establish adequate support, and set and declutter your path.

I advised Mary that only she can make appropriate choices. Each person must consider factors, such as health status, mobility, age, allergies, sensitivities, likes, and dislikes. For example, someone who has celiac disease must avoid foods with gluten, a person with back problems may need mild forms of exercise, and a person with unresolved sleep issues may need to consult with a sleep expert. For Mary to enjoy her new lifestyle, her choices must be sensible, sustainable, and pleasurable. To make informed choices, she required a basic understanding of how food affects the body. Thus, our discussion began with the following four food-related choices that are impactful to weight loss:

CLEAR CHOICES: FOOD

1. **Essential Nutrients:** understanding how whole foods and processed, nutrient-poor foods affect the body.

2. **Healthy Balance:** establishing a lifestyle grounded in proper portions of nourishing foods; while permitting small amounts of substances that do not serve the body well.

3. **Eating organic:** Reducing consumption of contaminated produce to lessen the potentially harmful effects on health and weight loss.

4. **Detoxification:** Eating clean, for a specific period to reduce the body's toxic load and aid in weight loss.

ESSENTIAL NUTRIENTS

I began by telling Mary that a client of mine once declared that food makes people sick. In reality, food is our life source. Flourish means to grow, develop well, or be healthy. For instance, a gardener might boast that his large, brightly colored vegetables are flourishing because of perfect weather conditions. Similar to plants that thrive on sunshine and water, the human body demands nutrients to stay healthy and alive.

So, I asked Mary, "What do you think would happen if you planted tomatoes in the shade and watered them once a month?" She paused; then said, "Most likely, they would fail to grow or become diseased." Mary was correct. Just like a tomato, your body cannot flourish without nutritious foods. To maintain health, Mary had to consume essential macronutrients and micronutrients. Especially, the phytonutrients found in fruits, vegetables, beans, nuts, seeds, whole grains, and other plant foods.

- Macronutrients are carbohydrates, proteins, and healthy fats. These are needed in more significant quantities to provide the body with energy.

- Micronutrients are vitamins and minerals. These are needed, every day, in smaller amounts for the body to properly function.

Conversely, nutrient-poor foods pack on the calories without providing the body with essential nutrients. Therefore, the body stores the unknown substances as fat to protect vital organs from harm. Examples of empty calorie foods include refined white flour and bread, donuts, cake, candy, table sugar, and soda. Often, vitamins and minerals are added to processed foods, such as cereals, because the natural nutrients are removed. The label claim on cereals and other processed foods with nutritional additives will indicate fortified.

Equally important, I advised Mary that eating too few calories, for her body size, might lead to malnutrition. Or, her metabolism might halt if she waits too long to eat between meals. In effect, the body "thinks" Mary is starving so it would store fat for future energy.

Because I brought up calorie intake, Mary asked if she needed to track everything she ate. I suggested that she log foods, for a few weeks, to recognize any connections between her eating patterns and emotions. That being said, a food diary can be helpful, but it is not essential to weight loss success. Over time, maintaining a healthy lifestyle becomes intuitive; instead of requiring an ongoing, time-consuming task. I emphasized that keeping a food diary is a personal choice. Calorie counting is less critical than choosing more quality, nutrient dense foods, and appropriate portions. On the other hand, Mary needed to learn how to balance her plate with healthy carbohydrates, fats, and protein.

HEALTHY BALANCE

Often, portion size relates to a specific food. For instance, a serving size of chicken or turkey is equivalent to a deck of cards or three ounces. However, the best way to illustrate balance is by viewing the contents of a healthy plate. The guideline below does not suggest that every meal will have the proposed combination of foods. Instead, Mary's target is to consume similar amounts of each food group throughout the day. For example, if she does not eat vegetables for breakfast, she might enjoy carrots with hummus for a snack.

I asked Mary to vision an average-sized plate filled with the following proportions of foods:

The left side of the plate:
- Three-quarters of vegetables and one-quarter of fruit.

The right side of the plate:
- Two-thirds of whole grains and one-third of protein.

Essential Add-ins:
- Healthy Fats: Such as olive oil, avocados, nuts, and nut butter.
- Water: Nine cups, average; unless prohibited by a health condition. The best indication that you are consuming enough water is clear urine color.

I recommended that Mary drink water before and after meals; not while eating. To clarify, the enzymes and acids in her stomach help to break down food. Drinking alkaline water while eating is like squirting a hose and extinguishing the necessary fire in the belly. As a result, adequate digestion of food and subsequent absorption might weaken.

After discussing portions with Mary, I gave her the following example plan to illustrate how to achieve a healthy balance throughout the day.

Breakfast:

- An omelet or scrambled eggs cooked with enough olive oil to coat the skillet. Choose between two whole eggs, one egg and two egg whites, or three egg whites.

- Add an ounce of diced, fresh mozzarella cheese and a favorite green vegetable, such as spinach, kale, or broccoli.

- Toast a slice of whole grain bread and top it with a tablespoon of apple butter or teaspoon of butter.

Lunch:

- A large salad made with salad greens, such as romaine, kale, arugula, endive, butterhead, baby spinach, green or red leaf lettuce.

- Toss in sweet vegetables or fruit or a combination of both. Vegetable suggestions are roasted butternut squash, carrots, or beets. Fruit suggestions are berries, sliced mango, pears, or orange wedges.

- Add in a protein, such as a tablespoon of chopped nuts or seeds. Alternatively, two to three ounces of diced chicken or turkey. Seed suggestions are pumpkin, sunflower, or hemp seeds.

- Dress with a light balsamic vinaigrette or drizzle with one tablespoon of olive oil and a fruit flavored vinaigrette.

Dinner:

- Lean meat, preferably chicken, turkey, salmon, other fish, beans, or tofu.

- Sweet potato, wild rice, brown rice, brown rice tortillas, whole grain pasta, corn, cornbread, quinoa, kasha, millet, buckwheat. Eat white potatoes and non-whole grain pasta in moderation.

- A non-starchy vegetable or combination, such as broccoli, asparagus, Brussel sprouts, spinach, mushrooms, artichoke hearts, cauliflower, okra, onions, zucchini, turnips, spaghetti squash, cucumber, tomatoes. If eating pasta, consider a side garden salad.

- Applesauce or fruit if two-three portions have not been eaten earlier in the day.

Snack examples for mid-morning and mid-afternoon:

- One ounce of nuts or a mixture of nuts and seeds.

- Plain fresh fruit or a tablespoon of peanut butter on apple slices or a small banana.

- A low sugar protein or granola bar; ideally, eight grams of sugar or less.

- Raw veggies, such as bell peppers, carrots, broccoli, cauliflower, or celery.

- An ounce of organic cheese paired with whole grain crackers.

- Organic plain yogurt topped with berries.

- Whole grain crackers or raw vegetables dipped in hummus or guacamole.

- Organic or popcorn made with three ingredients, corn, sea salt, olive oil.

- A small square of dark chocolate; preferably 70% or more cocoa.

Expectedly, Mary provided feedback on my sample meal plan. She asked for a quicker breakfast option because of her hectic morning schedule. So, I offered her a few alternatives. Specifically, Mary could prepare a dozen hard boiled eggs in advance. Then, she could conveniently pair a cooked egg with a slice of avocado and whole grain toast. Or, Mary might make an oatmeal bake or vegetable quiche, and enjoy a slice, each morning, with nuts and berries.

> *"... food is not simply organic fuel to keep body and soul together, it is a perishable art that must be savoured at the peak of perfection."*
>
> - E.A. Bucchianeri, Brushstrokes of a Gadfly

Also, I suggested that Mary experiment with different breakfast foods to see how she felt afterward. Although oatmeal is a healthy whole grain option, some people experience hunger within an hour because carbohydrates transform into sugar reasonably quick. Notably, a person's blood sugar level might spike; then, suddenly drop. When this happens, the body craves additional food. For this reason, paying attention to how your mood and body react to foods is essential to making choices that work for you. Hence, the plan that I provided is only intended to give guidance. To simplify how to achieve a healthy balance, I created an illustration that includes a list of recommended foods and substances to increase, decrease, and avoid.

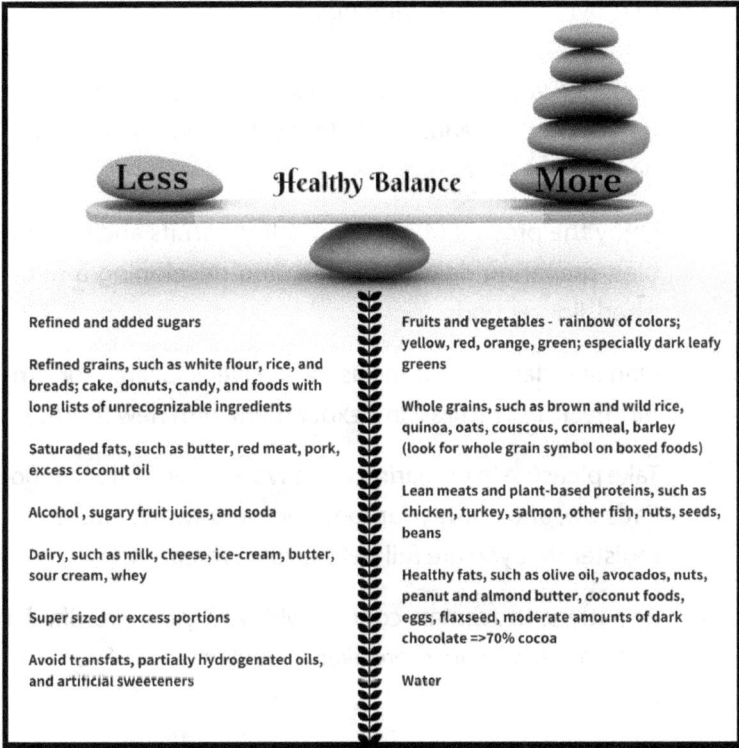

Less **Healthy Balance** **More**

Refined and added sugars	Fruits and vegetables - rainbow of colors; yellow, red, orange, green; especially dark leafy greens
Refined grains, such as white flour, rice, and breads; cake, donuts, candy, and foods with long lists of unrecognizable ingredients	
	Whole grains, such as brown and wild rice, quinoa, oats, couscous, cornmeal, barley (look for whole grain symbol on boxed foods)
Saturated fats, such as butter, red meat, pork, excess coconut oil	
	Lean meats and plant-based proteins, such as chicken, turkey, salmon, other fish, nuts, seeds, beans
Alcohol , sugary fruit juices, and soda	
Dairy, such as milk, cheese, ice-cream, butter, sour cream, whey	
	Healthy fats, such as olive oil, avocados, nuts, peanut and almond butter, coconut foods, eggs, flaxseed, moderate amounts of dark chocolate =>70% cocoa
Super sized or excess portions	
Avoid transfats, partially hydrogenated oils, and artificial sweeteners	Water

Next, I shared with Mary how to practice mindful eating. One element of mindfulness is to pause before deciding what to eat. For instance, recall what you ate for breakfast before choosing your next snack or meal. If your breakfast was high in protein, such as eggs or meat, then choose fresh fruit or carrots with hummus for a snack in lieu of a protein bar or nuts.

When I released the myths about dieting, I changed my mind-set and began treating healthy eating as an art. To explain, an artist is mindful in selecting paint colors, delights in painting, and carefully works to create the perfect image he or she has in mind. Thus, I suggested that Mary approach eating in the same manner. I provided the following tips:

- Connect with the idea that you are choosing quality foods for yourself. Schedule visits to local farmers' markets and health food stores.

- Enjoy the process of selecting colorful fruits and vegetables, preparing delicious meals, and developing a nourished, lighter body.

- Plan and design your meals for the week. Search for simple, healthier recipes and experiment with new foods.

- Take pleasure in preparing and savoring each bite of food. Eat slow, and chew your food thoroughly. Your mind will register that you are full before you overeat.

- Be patient and remain content with your progress. Similar to painting, you are more likely to feel pressure if you rush the activity.

- Celebrate and admire the masterpiece that you are designing.

Generally, I apply all of the Clear Lifestyle Practices; however, there are days, when I am off balance. For instance, during vacation, I look forward to savoring every bite of a restaurant quality cheeseburger. Sometimes, I pair it with a side salad and other times I choose crispy fries. Even so, I do not feel guilty. Remember, when you miss the bullseye it is because you permit yourself. When you stop beating yourself up over misses, you create a healthy relationship with food. It is important to realize that by eating more nutritious foods, you naturally crowd out the junk. A healthy balance requires choosing more whole foods, sensible portion sizes, and less processed non-foods.

*"It's important to have a healthy balanced diet
but not to get too bogged down in it.
It's important to enjoy your food, too."*

- Katie Taylor

Realizing that perfection is not part of a healthy lifestyle, Mary left our session feeling ready to move forward with improved eating habits.

Two weeks later, she entered my office beaming, again, because she shed another two pounds. After Mary shared her progress and gratifying experience at the gym, I introduced the topic of organic foods.

EATING ORGANIC

A point often overlooked is that toxin overload can cause weight loss plateaus. Pollutants and chemicals, such as pesticides, are found in many foods. Additionally, toxins are abundant in personal care products, alcohol, drugs, and the environment. In effect, Mary's detoxifying organs, such as the kidney and liver, might become overburdened. In that event, fat cells would surround the toxic substances to prevent them from injuring vital organs. Another critical point is that studies have revealed that pesticides stress the immune system and increase the risk of diseases, such as cancer.

*"Chronic disease is a foodborne illness.
We ate our way into this mess, and we must eat our way out."*

- Mark Hyman, M.D.

Because Mary consumed a lot of processed foods in the past, I encouraged her to reduce consumption of chemical-laden produce. Chiefly, her fat cells would begin to shrink as the toxin load lessened; thus, mitigating the chance of a developing a resistant weight loss plateau.

I advised her that organic crops are void of harmful pesticides, fertilizers, and herbicides. Furthermore, organic animal meats do not contain antibiotics and hormones commonly given to factory farmed cattle and chickens. Being that, Mary understood that she would be exposing her body to the same harmful substances contained in the foods she buys. Then, I shared information on organic trends to support my recommendation.

According to Organic Authority, "In 2016, the organic food market reached a whopping $43 billion, and organic food currently represents 5.3 percent of total retail food sales in the U.S."

"The demand for organic food is growing at a remarkable rate. Consumers have made it clear that they want organic produce and every sector of the food chain is responding, with the kind of results we have just seen."

- Prince Charles

In 2018, the Environmental Working Group released its new "Dirty Dozen" list of fruits and vegetables. The guide added hot peppers; thus, expanding from 12 to 13 foods containing the highest levels of pesticide residue.

Environmental Working Group's: 2018 Shopper's Guide to Pesticides in Produce™

1. Strawberries
2. Spinach
3. Nectarines
4. Apples
5. Grapes
6. Peaches
7. Cherries
8. Pears
9. Tomatoes
10. Celery
11. Potatoes
12. Sweet Bell Peppers
13. +Hot Peppers

I reviewed the above items with Mary and suggested that she shop around before making a Clear Choice about eating organic. Ultimately, she had to decide what is best for her health and budget. Without delay, Mary chose to purchase organic strawberries and grapes because she ate them frequently. Then, based on the cost, she planned on buying additional organic foods.

Undoubtedly, Mary's health and body size would improve naturally by eating more whole foods and less processed items. What must be remembered is that our bodies become increasingly vulnerable to illness as toxins accumulate and weaken our immune system.

"I would like to see people more aware of where their food comes from. I would like to see small farmers empowered. I feed my daughter almost exclusively organic food."

- Anthony Bourdain

Next, I asked Mary if she was open to hearing about an option to detoxify her body further. Without delay, she agreed.

DETOXIFICATION

In essence, detoxification is a time-limited elimination diet that enables the body to purge unhealthy toxins and wastes. The detox process reduces toxic burden on the body, aids in digestion, fortifies the immune system, and helps the body to heal naturally. Additionally, you learn how to eat clean while enhancing your health. For anyone who plans to begin a journey to renewed health, re-establishing the body's optimum state is an outstanding choice. In other words, you commit to cleansing your body of the toxic load and harmful effects; then, maintain a healthier lifestyle.

After I explained the goal of detoxification, Mary revealed

that she had once used a seven-day cleansing system to lose weight. I was pleased that she shared her experience so that I could further advise about safe detoxification. First, I reinforced that weight loss is a by-product of an elimination diet; not the intention. Second, a safe cleanse requires several weeks for proper metabolic processing. For example, the liver is the body's primary detoxifying organ. When the liver becomes overloaded, normal functioning is impaired. If Mary attempts to rid her body of harmful substances too fast, the toxins may release from fat cells and hang out in her body before the body can appropriately purge them. The liver needs time to convert the harmful substances into water-soluble nutrients. Hence, Mary could re-toxify her body. To emphasize, the reason that some women struggle to lose excess pounds is that fat cells hold on to toxins.

Thus, I explained the following elements for, both, safe and effective detoxification:

- Remove highly processed foods and replace them with whole organic foods. As best as possible, select foods that are free of additives, preservatives, pesticides, hormones, antibiotics, artificial sweeteners, and long lists of unrecognizable ingredients. By eating more conventionally grown fruits, vegetables, and other produce, you gain more energy and improve health by fueling the body with more nutrients.

- Eliminate common food allergens, such as gluten, dairy, soy, and refined sugars. You might be unaware of a connection between your health and foods that are known to cause an allergic immune response. By temporarily removing these foods from your diet, you might discover the triggers associated with headaches, skin problems, pain, bloating, inflammation, etc. Also, limiting sugar is essential to balancing your blood sugar level and losing weight.

- Eliminate or reduce consumption of acidic foods, such as alcohol, carbonated and sweetened beverages, pork, and vinegar-except for raw apple cider vinegar. Foods can range from highly acidic to alkalizing. Eating an abundance of acidic foods effects the body's pH levels and increases the risk of disease. A person can manage his or her pH balance by consuming more organic produce, water, and plant-based proteins, such as beans.

Also, According to Dr. Josh Axe, DNM, DC, CNS, "Limiting consumption of acid-forming foods and eating more alkaline-forming foods can protect your body from obesity by decreasing leptin levels and inflammation, which affects your hunger and fat-burning abilities. Since alkaline-forming foods are anti-inflammatory foods, consuming an alkaline diet gives your body a chance to achieve normal leptin levels and feel satisfied from eating the number of calories you really need."

After learning about detoxification, Mary expressed interest; however, she needed time think it over. I reminded her that I aim to provide food-related choices; not to prescribe a plan. A detox might seem overwhelming because of the temporary restrictions; however, I know it is an important option to share because my clients are happily amazed by the results.

Frankly, I wish someone had shared the benefits of detoxification when I embarked on my health journey. As previously mentioned, I had struggled with plateaus; especially midway to my weight loss goal. I had not purged my body of toxins, and I continued to consume foods made of chemicals, such as artificial sweeteners.

The results of my first detox were so surprising that I committed to repeating the process twice a year. I experienced a significant increase in energy, my sleep became quick and deep, and I shed the seven pounds gained after a lengthy, demobilizing foot injury. I felt healthier than I had ever been. Because of the health advantage, I offer detoxification to all of my clients. Accordingly, I let Mary know that I would happily guide her through this process at any point in her life.

Kiddingly, I told Mary to sleep on it. She chuckled and said, "I might have trouble with that recommendation because I am not sleeping well." Since the connection between sleep and weight is no laughing matter, I responded by giving her a handout on sleep tips to read before our next session. Also, I recommend that she complete the Clear Choices-Food Worksheet.

CLEAR CHOICES - FOOD WORKSHEET

Complete the worksheet below to document the food-related choices essential to:

- Increasing nutrient intake
- Establishing a healthy balance of carbohydrates, protein, and healthy fats
- Decreasing the toxic load on your body

Note: Carbohydrates, protein, and fats exist in a variety of foods. For instance, nuts are both a protein source and provide healthy fats.

I will increase my intake of nutrients by eating appropriate portions of the following foods:

- **Fresh or frozen fruits**

_____

_____

_____

- **Fresh or Frozen Vegetables,** including dark leafy greens and a variety of colorful produce

_____

_____

_____

Note: Both starchy and non-starchy vegetables contain healthy carbohydrates. Examples of high starch vegetables are corn, potatoes, peas, and sweet squash. To establish a healthy, balanced plate, reduce the frequency of eating two high starch vegetables during the same meal. For example, enjoy an ear of corn with grilled chicken and a garden salad.

- **Protein - plant-based sources:** Nuts, nut butter, beans, seeds, grains, and vegetables

_____

_____

_____

Note: High protein vegetable sources include, but are not limited to broccoli, spinach, peas, Brussel sprouts, kale, artichokes, mushrooms. Examples of high protein grains are quinoa, spelt, amaranth, and teff.

- **Protein - meat sources:** poultry, fish, pork, beef, eggs, other wild game, cheese, and other dairy products

_____

_____

_____

Note: Balance the consumption of plant and meat-based proteins throughout the day. Limit portions of foods that are highest in saturated fats, such beef and dairy products. Cheese and ice-cream are common-high sources of saturated fat. Select low-fat or naturally lower fat cheeses, such as Parmesan, Mozzarella, and Feta.

- **Healthy Fats:** Examples include, olive oil, avocados, nuts, peanut and almond butter, coconut foods, eggs, flaxseed, moderate amounts of dark chocolate =>70% cocoa

_____

_____

_____

Note: Healthy fats are important for proper bodily function.

Consider a quality Omega-3 supplement to enhance your intake; especially if you do not enjoy eating the foods listed above.

- **Whole Grains:** Examples include, brown and wild rice, brown rice tortillas and chips, quinoa, oats, whole wheat couscous, whole grain cornmeal, whole corn, whole wheat, barley, spelt, teff, and amaranth. When buying other boxed or bagged foods, look for the Whole Grain Symbol illustrated below.

_____

_____

_____

Note: Often, people who struggle to lose weight eat too many carbohydrates; especially pastries and refined grains, such as white flour, rice, breads, pasta, crackers, cereals, flour tortillas, pitas, etc. As a result, their body continuously burns excess carbohydrates for energy; instead of burning fat. Unlike white grains that are stripped of essential nutrients, whole grains maintain the outer bran layer and the core germ. These are the substances that are fiber-rich and contain vitamins, minerals, and healthy fats. About 50% of all carbohydrates consumed should be whole grains.

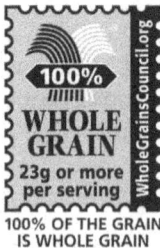

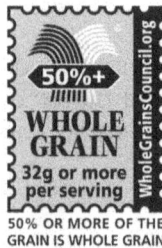

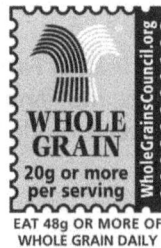

100% WHOLE GRAIN 23g or more per serving / WholeGrainsCouncil.org	**50%+** WHOLE GRAIN 32g or more per serving / WholeGrainsCouncil.org	WHOLE GRAIN 20g or more per serving / WholeGrainsCouncil.org
100% OF THE GRAIN IS WHOLE GRAIN	50% OR MORE OF THE GRAIN IS WHOLE GRAIN	EAT 48g OR MORE OF WHOLE GRAIN DAILY

I will decrease my intake of excess fats, sugars, chemicals, and other toxins by:

- **Consuming less of the following processed and empty calorie foods:**

_____

_____

_____

Because sugar in addictive and consumption of excess amounts affect blood sugar levels, fat storage, and overall health, limiting intake is imperative to weight loss and overall health.

Examples of empty calorie foods include: *candy, donuts, cake, pie, pastries, soda, sweets, artificial sweeteners, alcohol, shortening, margarine, soda, fruit and energy drinks, hot dogs, bacon, luncheon meats, pre-packaged microwaveable meals, white bread and rice, cereals, potato and corn chips*

- **Purchasing the following organic foods:**

_____

_____

_____

Note: Foods with the highest levels of pesticide residues are: Strawberries, spinach, nectarines, apples, grapes, peaches, cherries, pears, tomatoes, celery, potatoes, sweet bell peppers, hot peppers. Also consider purchasing organic grass-fed beef and poultry free of antibiotic and hormones.

"Not getting enough sleep is one of the strongest individual factors for weight gain and obesity"

- Clean Start Weight Loss®

CLEAR CHOICES: SLEEP

Pale yellow curtains seemed to dance to the gentle breeze that flowed through my office window. The room was comfortably cool despite the sun's warming rays. The pleasant morning inspired me to establish a calming atmosphere aligned with a planned discussion about the importance of sleep. So, I diffused a lavender scent into the air and turned on the soothing sound of contemporary instrumental music.

As a former night owl who averaged five hours of sleep per night, I made it a goal to learn how to achieve a good night's rest. Frankly, changing and maintaining better sleep habits took longer than losing my weight.

According to Harvard Medical School's Sleep Medicine Division, "Numerous studies have found that insufficient sleep increases a person's risk of developing serious medical conditions, including obesity, diabetes, and cardiovascular disease." Additionally, driving when your drowsy increases the risk of automobile accidents.

Because I was aware of Mary's struggles with stress-related emotional eating, I knew that her additional sleep issues could inadvertently sabotage her plan to eat healthier foods and maintain energy. The materials that I gave Mary, two weeks earlier, described the connection between inadequate slumber and weight.

As soon as I greeted Mary, she reported another one pound loss of body fat and showed me pictures of her new clothes. She was so excited and quick to share her progress that she had not noticed the ambiance of the room. Finally, the conversation paused, she sniffed the air and began humming to the music. We both laughed for a moment. Then, in a playful tone, she asked, "Are you trying to put me to sleep?"

When Mary told me that she did not return to the gym, I asked her why. She confessed that cooking and cleaning trumped exercising in the evenings when her energy level was high. As suspected, Mary could not sustain her energy by healthy eating alone. After we reviewed the sleep topics below, Mary recognized habits that needed to change. As usual, I recommended that she complete the corresponding Clear Choices - Sleep Worksheet. Furthermore, I suggested that we talk more about exercise. Although Mary had chosen to join a fitness center, I wanted her to consider various forms of physical activity to increase the likely hood of sustaining a program that she would enjoy.

Effects of Inadequate Sleep

- Like stress, sleep deprivation produces higher levels of cortisol and activates the hunger hormone, ghrelin. As previously mentioned, cortisol causes the fight or flight response. As a result, your body craves food to make you feel better and provide energy; typically, carbohydrates and fats. In other words, lack of sleep increases your appetite and triggers the reward system in your brain. Consequently, you eat to release serotonin, a chemical that regulates your mood and other physical and mental functions.

- Lack of rest slows down your metabolism and results in increased insulin production. These factors combined with an elevated cortisol level stimulates the body to store calories as fat. Equally important, researchers at the University of Chicago, found that lack of sleep substantially decreases insulin sensitivity, the cause of increased production. Over time, the excess fat is stored in organs, such as the liver; resulting in diabetes and other chronic conditions.

- Your body produces lower levels of leptin. This hormone is produced in your fats cells and keeps the stomach feeling full. The less leptin your body makes, the more hungry you become. Together with the increase in cortisol, ghrelin, and insulin, you will struggle to control your appetite and make healthy food choices.

- When you are overtired, you are more inclined to eat unhealthy fast or take out foods instead of cooking at home.

- Lack of adequate rest and a low energy level leads to physical inactivity. Thus, you burn fewer calories.

- According to the National Sleep Foundation, "…women who sleep five hours or less a night are 15 percent more likely to become obese over the course of 16 years than those who sleep for at least seven hours."

"Sleep is important as a major component of good health. A lack of sleep, or a poor quality of sleep, can sabotage a person's health goals and impair their safety. Many patients would have had to spend less time in a hospital or ER if they discovered the importance of a good night's sleep. We tend to treat sleep as a health non-entity instead of a vital component of a healthy lifestyle. It is past time that the medical community "wakes people up" to the importance of a proper amount and quality of sleep. This will make our patients healthier, and our roads safer."

- Brendan Duffy

In the event that you become short of breath, frequently and suddenly wake during sleep, snore loudly, develop headaches, or feel extremely tired or irritable during the day, you may have sleep apnea. Obesity can cause this serious sleep disorder, a condition that disrupts breathing throughout the night. Some forms of sleep apnea result from the excess soft tissue that forms in the neck and mouth. If you experience these symptoms, the best intervention is to seek medical advice.

Ways to Assess and Improve Sleep Hygiene

- **Get on a schedule**: Your body sleeps best at night when it is dark. It also functions best when you keep a routine. Plan to go to bed at the same time each evening and awake at the same time every morning. According to Dr. James Maass, author of *Sleep for Success* and *Power Sleep,* "If you stick to a schedule, your body is more alert than if you sleep for the same total amount of time at varying hours during the week."

- **Practice a relaxing bedtime ritual:** Prepare your body for the transition from a busy day to a long night of rest. Engage in a calming activity, such as reading or meditation.

- **Evaluate your room:** Design your sleep environment to establish the conditions you need for sleep. Your bedroom should be cool, between 60-67 degrees, and free from any noise that can disturb your sleep. Your bedroom should be free from light and disruptions, such as a snoring partner. Consider using blackout shades or curtains, an eye mask, or earplugs.

- **Sleep on a comfortable mattress and pillows:** Life expectancy for most good quality mattresses is nine to ten years. If yours has exceeded life expectancy, you may need to replace it for comfort and support. Make the room attractive and inviting to sleep, but also free of allergens. Use calming colors to decorate the room.

- **Avoid naps:** If you struggle to fall or stay asleep, avoid naps. However, when fatigue sets in, a quick nap can do wonders for your mental and physical stamina. A short rest, 20-30 minutes, provides significant benefit for improved alertness and performance without leaving you feeling groggy or interfering with nighttime sleep. Keep in mind that getting regular, adequate sleep helps you feel your best and stay alert.

- **Use light to manage your body rhythms:** If you are exposing yourself to artificial, electric light, from computers or other devices, it may be interfering with your ability to sleep. The light coming from the screens of these devices is activating your brain. Avoid electronics at least 30 minutes before bed and in the middle of the night.

- **Avoid alcohol, cigarettes, caffeine, and heavy meals in the evening:** Alcohol, cigarettes, and caffeine can disrupt sleep. Eating big and spicy meals can cause discomfort and indigestion that can make it hard to sleep. Try to stop eating at least two hours before bedtime. Eat a light, healthy snack if you are hungry in the evening.

- **Exercise daily:** Vigorous exercise is best, but some light movement is better than no activity. Exercise any time of day, but not at the expense of your sleep.

- **Eat Healthy:** Sustaining a healthy diet supports weight loss and aids in improving sleep. To mitigate sleep disruptions, reduce the amount of fluids you drink before bedtime. Also, eat a filling breakfast to prevent a ravenous appetite, excess snacking, and overeating later in the day.

CLEAR CHOICES - SLEEP WORKSHEET

Complete the worksheet below to assess your sleep hygiene and choose areas to change or improve habits for healthier sleep.

1. **I maintain a consistent sleep schedule; striving to sleep at least seven hours**

   _____

   _____

2. **I have established a relaxing bedtime ritual**

   _____

   _____

3. **My sleep environment is cool, free of noise, and dark**

   _____

   _____

4. **My mattress and pillows are comfortable**

   _____

   _____

5. **I avoid naps. However, when I'm fatigued, I take a short 20-30 minute nap to refresh myself**

   _____

   _____

6. I avoid electronics, such as televisions, phones, and computers at least 30 minutes before bedtime

_____

_____

7. I avoid alcohol, cigarettes, caffeine, and heavy meals in the evening

_____

_____

8. I exercise daily - includes light physical activity such as walking

_____

_____

9. I plan to seek medical attention for symptoms related to sleep apnea

_____

_____

"Movement is a medicine for creating change in a person's physical, emotional, and mental state."

- Carol Welch

CLEAR CHOICES: PHYSICAL ACTIVITY

Typically, I wear casual business clothes when meeting with a client in person. However, I surprised Mary by dressing in comfortable fitness wear for our session. My goal was to demonstrate a few simple home exercises instead of explaining them. She suggested that I don this same attire for future meetings to inspire her. I looked directly into Mary's eyes and stated, "The most powerful inspiration lies within you. By practicing the Clear Lifestyle Practices that you have learned, you have the power to be unstoppable." Mary sheepishly grinned; then replied, I know. I have to train my mind to believe in myself. Straightaway, I asked her what had gone well over the past two weeks.

I was delighted to hear that Mary had returned to the gym four times since we last met. Mary attributed her progress to improved sleep and feeling lighter. By reducing caffeine intake and eliminating her evening glass of wine, she slept through the night and no longer felt tired and anxious during the day. Additionally, she downsized another pound. Next, I asked if she intended to increase her physical activity level since she established a goal to exercise at least five times per week. After an uncomfortable period of silence, she said, "Yes," but, I don't think I'll be going to the fitness center more than three times each week." Then, I asked her, "What activity did you enjoy most at the gym?" Mary replied, "The stationary bicycle and the treadmill." Next, I inquired, "Do you think that you would find pleasure in walking or riding a bike around your neighborhood?" She immediately answered, "I've been thinking about buying a bike." I encouraged Mary to make the purchase and reflect on activities that brought pleasure to her in the past. I shared that listening to music motivates me to get up and walk, dance, clean, cook, and work in the yard.

According to Jeanette Bicknell, PhD., "Listening to music during exercise can both delay fatigue and lessen the subjective perception of fatigue. It can increase physical capacity, improve energy efficiency, and influence mood. In study after study, the use of music during low-to moderate-level intensity exercise was associated with clear improvements in endurance."

I emphasized that keeping her body in motion is essential to sustained weight loss and health. Then we discussed that lack of physical activity is a primary cause of most chronic diseases. People who have an inactive lifestyle:

- Burn fewer calories; increasing the likelihood of gaining weight.
- Slow down metabolism; the body might have trouble breaking down fats and sugars
- Lose muscle strength and endurance because the muscles are not used enough
- Weaken the bones and lose some mineral content
- Effect how well the immune system functions

- Have poorer blood circulation
- Increase chances of inflammation
- Develop hormonal imbalance
- Might cause digestive issues and constipation

Equally important, I recommended that Mary schedule activities during the time of day when she is most energetic. Also, I provided several examples to clarify what qualifies as a movement:

- Stretching
- Walking up and down stairs
- Walking in malls
- Brisk walking outside or on a treadmill
- Parking her vehicle a distance away from the office
- Cleaning the house
- Working in the garden
- Riding a bike, swimming or other sports
- Dancing
- Sit-ups
- Squats
- Leg presses
- Lifting weights
- Running

Then, I sprung from my chair and grabbed a box of at-home exercise equipment. I mentioned that I begin my day with a 12 minute guided yoga routine to stretch all of my muscles. When

I am at the gym, I warm up on the treadmill before engaging in strength training. According to the American College of Sports Medicine, "Flexibility prepares the muscles, tendons, and joints for work by allowing them to move freely through a full active range of motion. The more prepared the body is, the less likely it is to get injured."

Accordingly, I encouraged Mary to pay attention to her body and develop a program suitable to her likes and comfort level. For example, someone with a back injury or arthritis may be able to tolerate swimming, but not lifting weights. I reminded her to speak with her physician before committing to any new exercises; especially those that put stress on the body.

After I recommended that Mary complete the Clear Choices-Fitness Worksheet, I proceeded to demonstrate the use of a resistance tube to tone my arms and shoulders. Mary also practiced a few movements and liked the ease of use. Next, I showed her how to use a soft medicine ball to strengthen her abdominal muscles. Lastly, I did three floor exercises that tone legs without the need for equipment. Afterward, I shared a humbling experience that taught me the importance of staying consistent with a fitness routine.

For three years, I faithfully worked out. I walked for four miles several times a week and spent alternate days toning my muscles at the gym. Then, I shattered the bone in my big toe, underwent surgery, and became immobile for six months. However, there was no reason to neglect my upper body. Nevertheless, I created a pity party for myself that extended beyond my ability to work-out. When I returned to exercise, I discovered that I had lost everything that I had gained. My knee became swollen during walks, and I could not lift the 10-pound dumbbells that I had previously raised, above my head, with ease. Even more disappointing, I struggled to lift 5-pound weights. One year later, I regained my strength and former abilities. I felt joyful about the accomplishment and promised myself never to let that happen again.

Now, reflect for a moment to consider the plight of people with disabilities who wish they could move differently, become athletes, or find a way to keep fit. So, no matter your size or circumstances there is always some form of physical activity that is suitable to your body; even if you are doing something while sitting in a chair. To emphasize, I could barely walk up steps without losing my breath when I weighed 242 pounds. I started slow, and I never gave up.

Every person needs to find something that he or she loves to do. I prefer walking in nature to take in the beauty that surrounds us. Sometimes I walk at a fast pace and other times I stroll to capture colorful pictures of flowers, trees, birds, and sunsets. In the colder months, I work out at home and visit the gym more often. Also, I became aware that my mood toward exercise improved once I invested in comfortable fitness clothes and sneakers.

"If you always put limits on everything you do, physical or anything else. It will spread into your work and into your life. There are no limits. There are only plateaus, and you must not stay there, you must go beyond them."

- Bruce Lee

To develop an exercise routine that fits your likes and lifestyle, complete the Clear Choices - Physical Activity Worksheet.

CLEAR CHOICES - PHYSICAL ACTIVITY WORKSHEET

Complete the worksheet below to choose the frequency, type(s), and method of accountability for establishing a fitness program.

I plan on exercising the same time of day to establish a routine (Yes/No) _____

I plan to track my movement for at least _____(days/weeks/months). **My reason is:**

_____

_____

_____

The best time of day for me to workout is _____
My reason is:

_____

_____

_____

The types of activity that I would enjoy and would be the easiest to maintain are:

_____

_____

_____

I plan to purchase a one or more pieces of equipment to exercise at home: (Yes/No) _____ My reason is:

_____

_____

_____

Examples of home equipment: Dumbbells, Resistance tubes or bands, Kettle ball, Medicine ball, Exercise or yoga mat, Jump rope, Ankle weights, Treadmill, Bike, Step, Pedometer for tracking steps.

Reflection for the Journey Ahead

I remember a time when I accepted and defended being overweight. I enjoyed my life and did not realize how much happier I could be by nourishing my mind, body, and spirit.

Our minds play a critical role in weight loss, but we feed it with limiting beliefs, doubt, negative thoughts, and dieting myths. On top of that, stress, emotions, and excess sugar trigger hormones and chemicals that influence our appetite, mood, choices, and health.

To win the battle with weight, women need to embrace a journey toward habit change. The path is happily traveled when practice and patience come along. For this reason, the Clear Lifestyle Practices are intended to be learned behaviors over time. The more you practice, the easier positive thoughts and habits transform into a natural part of your lifestyle. The bottom line is that the journey never ends. The Road ahead will help you to learn, grow, and achieve your goals. However, the practices must be sustained throughout life to maintain what you have accomplished. In like manner, a house requires upkeep after you pay the mortgage in full.

Reflecting on the Clear Lifestyle Practices

You step onto a path that is designed by you. You stand still for a moment, smile, take a deep breath, and close your eyes. You feel powerful and relaxed because you chose to be the boss of your life. You own the business of enhancing your health. Nobody has the authority to rule your choices or actions. You developed a strategic plan to lead your life to a destination so beautiful that you will never want to go back to where you started. Your objectives of your journey include:

1. **Develop a Clear Why:** Business leaders determine the reason for a new program, product, or service. They aim to fulfill someone's demand. Therefore, you must create a why for weight loss that aligns with what you feel you need to be successful. You mindfully recall your why, as necessary, to trigger internal motivation.

2. **Establish Clear Goals:** Documented milestones and targets measure progress and success. Periodically check your status; however, focus on the actions that lead to the outcome. Do not obsess over the data point because it will not change without effort. If your compass reflects that you are off the path, then re-align your habits in the direction of your destination. Refrain from feelings of guilt when you miss the target. Be patient, stay positive, and take another step forward.

3. **Arrange Clear Support:** Intelligent leaders surround themselves with positive people who reinforce their path, provide assistance, and celebrate successes. They know that there will be people who will not agree with their

plan, make negative comments, and attempt to impede progress. Likewise, you might face the same challenges. To keep your spirit nourished, make sure that you have at least one like-minded person who will happily lend an ear, a heart, or a hand.

4. **Design a Clear Path:** Executives do not accept excuses. Instead, they expect a plan to remove or mitigate the barriers that obstruct achievement of goals and objectives. Lack of time is a common obstacle to healthy activities, such as cooking and exercise. As the boss, you are in charge of removing the barriers that might hinder achievement of your goals. Become intentional about how you spend the 24 hours in each day.

5. **Frame a Clear Vision:** Business strategy addresses what needs to happen now and in the future. Chiefs know that change is inevitable, so they imagine what lies ahead. In like manner, by forming and a mental picture of your desired state, you stay focused on where you are going and not where you are now. Your objective is to recall your why; then frame it with an image of your future self. In effect, you have the power to manifest what your mind sees into reality.

6. **Form a Clear Mind:** A wise leader inspires hope and fosters a positive outlook. Any sensible person who manages people knows that cultivating a negative culture demotivate staff and increases the chance of failure. Because you are leading yourself, success necessitates that you pay attention to how you feel. Once you recognize what caused a negative emotion, you can shift your thoughts

to something positive. Consequently, the choices that you make are a direct reflection of your mood. Because behavior is vital to weight loss, you have to consciously shape your attitude by using your mind as a tool. Additionally, reflective and spiritual practices help to calm and clear the mind.

7. **Own Clear Choices:** Executives are responsible for outcomes. Sometimes they ask for input on a topic or project, but, ultimately, the decision rests in their hands. In the same fashion, you are accountable for the choices you make related to food, sleep, and physical activity.

At the start of your journey, change is challenging because your body is likely working against you. For instance, you may crave sugar because of the types of foods that you have eaten in the past. Additionally, hormones, biological chemicals, and toxins may be affecting your hunger, mood, and feelings of discomfort. For this reason, you need to use your mind to make deliberate choices. Slow down, take a deep breath, and pause before making a choice. Tell yourself that you can; then recall your why, picture your future, enlist support when needed, and think about your body as a work of art. Continue to remove or fix the obstacles that arise along your path.

As you break the cycle of sugar addition and implement practices to improve sleep, increase movement, and eat healthier, the journey becomes easier and enjoyable. Never forget how powerful your mind is to your success. Lead your life feeling empowered to make changes that lessen your busyness. Consciously, shift worries and negative thoughts to hope, faith, and gratitude.

Make time for self care. Let go of the belief that dieting is the answer. Remember that a diet represents the type of foods you eat, thus it can be healthy or unhealthy.

Your health is the most crucial possession in your life; therefore, you deserve to know what is necessary to manage weight throughout life. Thus, the placement of Clear Choices at the end of this book is intentional.

First, I aimed to empower you with customizable lifestyle practices designed to set you up for long-term success. Then, I guided you with choices that are vital to achieving a sustainable, healthy weight.

In conclusion, a healthy and happier lifestyle encompasses mental, emotional, spiritual, and physical well-being. Each of these areas are interconnected; thus you must work on them simultaneously to produce the healthier body and lifestyle that you deserve.

"Life is a journey, and only you hold the map."

- CoolSmart.com

Destined to Be Healthy
- Time to Take the Wheel

Tomorrow is a promising start to my brand new year

To make it my best, I'm grabbing hold of the gear

I'm ready to shift from idle park into active drive

I'm headed to a healthier place to feel more alive

Here, I'm comfortable, but I could have more fun

So, I've decided to walk, dance, or maybe I'll run

I'll need high quality fuel, the energy I need to get there

I'll choose healthier, fresh, whole foods because I care

My engine will have more power by replacing all the junk

I'm sure to reach my destination because I've got the spunk

I'll plan for plenty of rest stops along the way

To recharge my battery so I'll conquer each day

I'm done being the passenger; just enjoying the view

I'll be the important driver for it's my destiny to choose

The size and shape of my vehicle I know matters not

I'll just step on the pedal and give it all that I've got

Actually, tomorrow is a promising start to a brand new me

I know the best route. It leads to the healthiest I can be

- Michele J. Rossi

About the Author

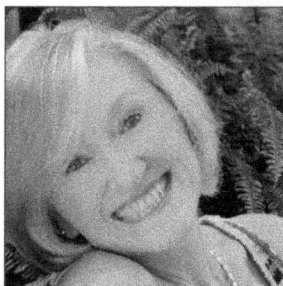

Michele J. Rossi is the CEO and Founder of Make Healthy Fit, Inc. and holds certifications as an Integrative Nutrition Health Coach and Training Facilitator. Michele became a health coach after her triumph over obesity and Type 2 diabetes. Determined to avoid insulin, she paved a new path to weight loss, shed 115 pounds, reversed her insulin resistance, ditched medications, and underwent excess skin removal surgery.

Michele serves as a speaker, private coach, leads group coaching programs, and health and wellness workshops. Her clients have achieved goals related to weight loss, blood sugar balance, stress reduction, energy levels, and harmony in all areas of life, including relationships.

In her pursuit to be an example of complete health, Michele merges her expertise in health coaching, dietary theories, and nutrition with experience and compassion to develop client-focused programs. She guides, advocates for; and empowers women to lead extraordinary lives by nourishing their mind, body, and spirit.

Before founding her own company, Michele held corporate leadership positions in large healthcare organizations. As a Certified Healthcare Quality Professional, she was responsible for educating and leading all levels of leadership, medical professionals, and staff to improve quality, patient safety, customer satisfaction, and compliance with accreditation and regulatory standards. Michele has served as the President of the Delaware Association for Healthcare Quality and a Judge among those who bestow the Delaware Quality Award for business.

Michele received her health coach training from the Institute for Integrative Nutrition and holds professional memberships with the International Association for Health Coaches, the American Diabetes Association, and International Association for Women.

Don't Miss a Thing!

Sign up for Michele's bi-weekly newsletter to receive health and wellness tips and mouth-watering recipes. https://michele-jazzalyn.com/newsletter

You can follow Michele on:

Instagram - https://www.instagram.com/healthjazz/
Facebook - https://www.facebook.com/MakeHealthyFit/
Pinterest - https://www.pinterest.com/makehealthyfit/
Twitter - https://twitter.com/MakeHealthyFit
LinkedIn - https://www.linkedin.com/in/makehealthyfit/

References

American Psychological Association. (n.d.). Making lifestyle changes that last. Retrieved from http://www.apa.org/helpcenter/life-style-changes.aspx

Baker, A., CN, LE. (2015, May 12). What happens when you detox? Retrieved April 10, 2018, from http://nourishholisticnutrition.com/what-happens-when-you-detox/

Bornstein, A. (2017, November 28). Why Sleep Is More Important Than We Ever Thought. Retrieved May 2, 2018, from https://www.shape.com/lifestyle/mind-and-body/why-sleep-no-1-most-important-thing-better-body

Burchard, B. (2017). High Performance Habits. Hay House.

Centers for Disease Control and Prevention. (2015, November). Adult Obesity Facts. Retrieved November 20, 2017, from https://www.cdc.gov/obesity/data/adult.html

E. M. (2018, January 16). The 9 Organic and Sustainable Food Trends Taking Over 2018. Retrieved April 8, 2018, from http://www.organicauthority.com/plant-based-and-more-on-the-rise-9-food-trends-to-watch-out-for-in-2018/

Harvard T.H. Chan School of Public Health. (2017, May 8). Doctors need more nutrition education. Retrieved from https://www.hsph.harvard.edu/news/hsph-in-the-news/doctors-nutrition-education/

Health Fitness Revolution. (2018, April 28). Top 10 Health Benefits of Journaling. Retrieved May 2, 2018, from http://www.healthfit-nessrevolution.com/top-10-health-benefits-journaling/

Institute for Integrative Nutrition®. (2013, 2016). *Are You Craving Movement* [PDF]. New York: Integrative Nutrition

Institute for Integrative Nutrition®. (2013, 2016). *Primary Foods* [PDF]. New York: Integrative Nutrition

Institute for Integrative Nutrition®. (2013, 2016). *U.S. Dietary Icons* [PDF]. New York: Integrative Nutrition.

J. A., DNM, DC, CNS. (n.d.). Is an Alkaline Diet the Key to Longevity? Retrieved May 5, 2018, from https://draxe.com/alkaline-diet/

J. B., Ph.D. (2013, January 30). Music and Exercise: What Current Research Tells Us. Retrieved April 28, 2018, from https://www.psychologytoday.com/us/blog/why-music-moves-us/201301/music-and-exercise-what-current-research-tells-us

Mayo Clinic. (2018, March 09). Sleep apnea. Retrieved May 2, 2018, from https://www.mayoclinic.org/diseases-conditions/sleep-apnea/symptoms-causes/syc-20377631

Maas, J. B., & Wherry, M. L. (2001). Power sleep: The revolutionary program that prepares your mind for peak performance. New York: Quill/HarperCollins.

M. D., MA, ATC. (2016, October 7). Basic Injury Prevention Concepts. Retrieved April 03, 2018, from http://www.acsm.org/public-information/articles/2016/10/07/basic-injury-prevention-concepts

M. J., Ph.D. (2017, September 28). Weight Loss and Sleep: Is There a Connection? Retrieved May 02, 2018, from https://www.psychologytoday.com/us/blog/sleep-newzzz/201709/weight-loss-and-sleep-is-there-connection-1

National Center for Complementary and Integrative Health. (2017, September 07). Meditation: In Depth. Retrieved from https://nccih.nih.gov/health/meditation/overview.htm

National Sleep Foundation. (2014, November 10). How Sleep Impacts Your Diet and Weight. Retrieved April 27, 2018, from https://sleep.org/articles/link-between-sleep-weight/

Psychology Today, C. R., Ph.D. (2014, June 23). 5 Scientifically Supported Benefits of Prayer. Retrieved from http://graceepiscopalchurch.org/wp-content/uploads/2016/10/science-prayer.pdf

Sifferlin, A. (2017, May 25). The Weight Loss Trap: Why Your Diet Isn't Working.Retrieved March 2, 2018, from http://time.com/magazine/us/4793878/] june-5th-2017-vol-189-no-21-u-s/

University of Minnesota, Taking Charge of Your Health and Well-being. (n.d.). What Is Spirituality? Retrieved April 8, 2018, from https://www.takingcharge.csh.umn.edu/what-spirituality

Wolf Management Consultants. (n.d.). Creating a Clear Vision of the Future. Retrieved April 25, 2018, from http://www.wolfmotivation.com/programs/creating-a-clear-vision-of-the-future

Wycklendt, M. (2015, March 17). Six reasons you'd be happier if you stopped saying "busy". Retrieved March 5, 2018, from https://www.washingtonpost.com/news/inspired-life/wp/2015/03/17/six-reasons-why-you-shouldnt-use-the-b-word-so-much/?noredirect=on&utm_term=.018fe7683df6

Resources

Michele J. Rossi
www.mj-rossi.com
Office: 609-202-8093
coach@mj-rossi.com

Hire Michele to Speak, Coach, or Train

- Seminars

- Health and wellness workshops

- One-on-one health coaching

- Workshops
  - Weigh Less for Life
  - Type 2 Diabetes - Reversing Insulin Resistance
  - Stress Less - Spiritual Path to Balance and Harmony
  - Conquering Sugar and Other Nagging Cravings
  - Wrap Yourself in Healthy Skin
  - 30 Days to Healthy Living; Detoxification Support
  - Customized Programs

Michele has been speaking to groups and organizations for 30+ years on health and wellness topics. She has coached groups, led workshops, and helped clients achieve goals related to weight and blood sugar management, stress reduction, increased energy levels, and achieve harmony in all areas of life, including relationships.

Institute for Integrative Nutrition

This book was inspired by my experience at the Institute for Integrative Nutrition® (IIN), where I received my training in holistic wellness and health coaching.

IIN offers a truly comprehensive Health Coach Training Program that invites students to deeply explore the things that are most nourishing to them. From the physical aspects of nutrition and eating wholesome foods that work best for each individual person, to the concept of Primary Food – the idea that everything in life, including our spirituality, career, relationships, and fitness contributes to our inner and outer health – IIN helped me reach optimal health and balance. I gained a deeper understanding of the interconnectedness of mind, body, and spirit. This inner journey unleashed the passion that compels me to share what I've learned and inspire others.

Beyond personal health, IIN offers training in health coaching, as well as business and marketing. Students who choose to pursue this field professionally complete the program equipped with the communication skills and branding knowledge they need to create a fulfilling career encouraging and supporting others in reaching their own health goals.

From renowned wellness experts as Visiting Teachers to the convenience of their online learning platform, this school has changed my life, and I believe it will do the same for you. I invite you to learn more about the Institute for Integrative Nutrition and explore how the Health Coach Training Program can help you transform your life. Feel free to contact me to hear more about my personal experience at www.mj-rossi.com or call (844) 315-8546 to learn more.

Acknowledgements

To my daughter, Sara, for her unconditional love and support throughout my lifestyle and career transformations. You inspire me to reach for the stars because I have watched you chase your dreams with a plan. You are my pride and joy. I love you.

To the Registered Dietician, Shannon Heffern, who coached me, a physically challenged women, through an extraordinary health transformation. Your compassionate and uplifting approach has influenced, both, the quality of my life and health coaching practice.

To the Fitness Coach, Lara Krygier, who challenged me with tough workout routines that helped to re-shape my body. Thank you for the reminder that my ultimate test of success is to hold myself accountable during your absence.

To my siblings, Ray, Brian, Theresa, and Dawn, for the bonds and beautiful memories that we have shared throughout our lives.

To the Salem County Commission on Women for recognizing and honoring my volunteer services. I am thankful for the opportunity to participate in strengthening our community through education and support.

A special thanks to my friends, Sandie Dyling and Jill Serubo, who have volunteered their time to help promote my business, Make Healthy Fit, Inc. I am grateful for your kindness and assistance.

To the extraordinary friend who served as my truth teller, pusher, and lifter so that I may serve my purpose by getting out of my comfort zone. Although you prefer to remain nameless, your gifts will remain tattooed in my heart and mind. Thank you for pointing me in the direction of my dream to live an extraordinary life by helping others to achieve success.

www.ingramcontent.com/pod-product-compliance
Lightning Source LLC
Chambersburg PA
CBHW050133280326
41933CB00010B/1366